MW01012128

LL COOL J's
PLATINUM 360
DIET AND LIFESTYLE

A FULL-CIRCLE GUIDE TO DEVELOPING YOUR MIND, BODY, AND SOUL

L L COOL J

WITH DAVID "SCOOTER" HONIG,
CHRIS PALMER, AND JIM STOPPANI, PhD

RODALE

This book is intended as a reference volume only, not as a medical manual.
The information given here is designed to help you make informed decisions about your health.
It is not intended as a substitute for any treatment that may have been prescribed by your doctor.
If you suspect that you have a medical problem, we urge you to seek competent medical help.

The information in this book is meant to supplement, not replace, proper exercise training.
All forms of exercise pose some inherent risks. The editors and publisher advise readers to take full
responsibility for their safety and know their limits. Before practicing the exercises in this book, be sure
that your equipment is well-maintained, and do not take risks beyond your level of experience, aptitude,
training, and fitness. The exercise and dietary programs in this book are not intended as a substitute
for any exercise routine or dietary regimen that may have been prescribed by your doctor. As with
all exercise and dietary programs, you should get your doctor's approval before beginning.

Mention of specific companies, organizations, or authorities in this book does not imply
endorsement by the author or publisher, nor does mention of specific companies, organizations,
or authorities imply that they endorse this book, its author, or the publisher.

Internet addresses and telephone numbers given in this book were accurate at the time it went to press.

© 2010 by James Todd Smith

All rights reserved. No part of this publication may be reproduced or transmitted in any form or by any means,
electronic or mechanical, including photocopying, recording, or any other information storage and retrieval system,
without the written permission of the publisher.

Rodale books may be purchased for business or promotional use or for special sales. For information, please write to:
Special Markets Department, Rodale Inc., 733 Third Avenue, New York, NY 10017

Printed in the United States of America
Rodale Inc. makes every effort to use acid-free ∞, recycled paper ♲.

Lifestyle and exercise photographs © 2010 by Scott McDermott
Food photographs © 2010 by Kate Mathis
Book design by Christopher Rhoads

Library of Congress Cataloging-in-Publication Data

LL Cool J.
    [Platinum 360 diet and lifestyle]
    LL Cool J's platinum 360 diet and lifestyle : a full-circle guide to developing your mind, body, and soul / LL Cool
J with David "Scooter" Honig . . . [et al.].
       p.   cm.
    Includes index.
    ISBN-13 978-1-60529-541-1 hardcover
    ISBN-10 1-60529-541-8 hardcover
    1. Physical fitness. 2. Exercise—Psychological aspects. 3. Diet. I. Title. II. Title: Platinum 360 diet and
lifestyle.
    RA781.L56 2010
    613.7'12—dc22
                                                                                2010001327

Distributed to the trade by Macmillan

2 4 6 8 10 9 7 5 3 1 hardcover

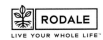

RODALE
LIVE YOUR WHOLE LIFE™

We inspire and enable people to improve their lives and the world around them
For more of our products visit **rodalestore.com** or call 800-848-4735

This book is dedicated to Scooter's mom, Frances.
Your toughness rubbed off on him
and his toughness truly helped me.
—LL COOL J

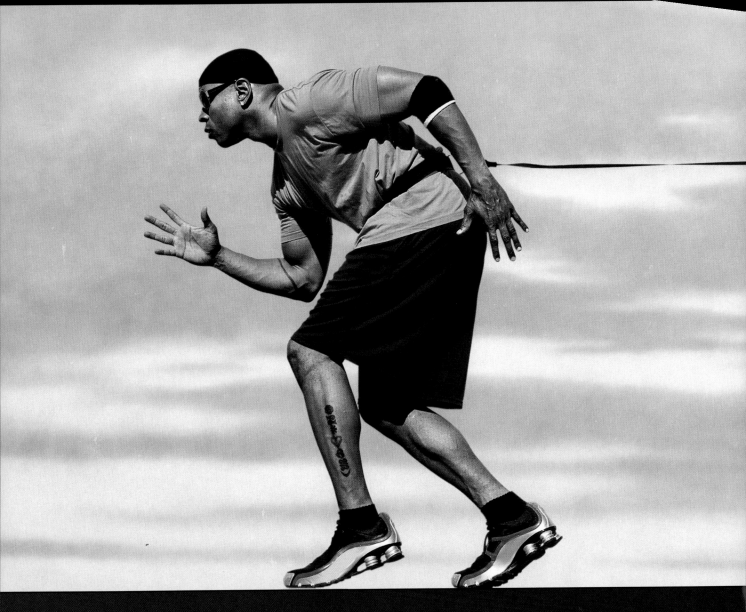

CONTENTS

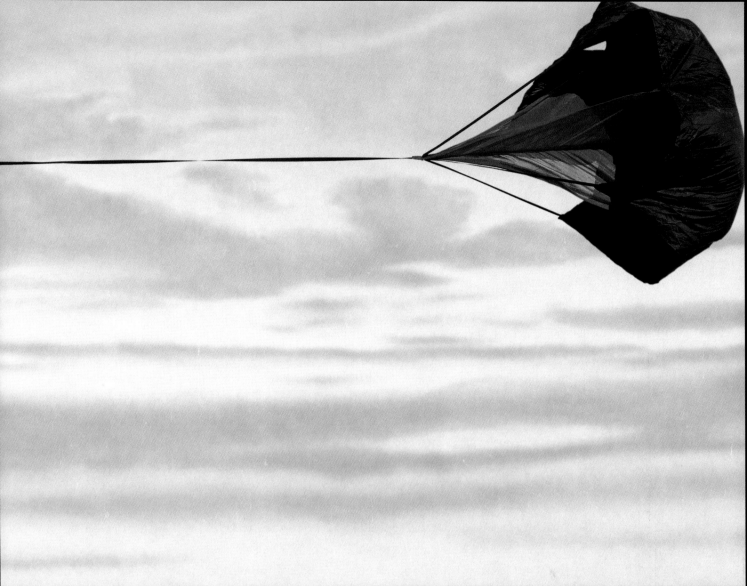

PART THREE
THE PLATINUM 360
NUTRITION PLAN

INTRODUCTION

It all starts with a simple question: Who am I? Rapper? Actor? Father? Son? Fitness buff? There was a time in my life when I could have answered that question without hesitation, delivering a well-rehearsed line from any talk-show couch or red-carpet lineup. My response would have been one or all of the above options.

Then a funny thing happened: I got a little older. I began to realize that as a younger man, I thought I had the answer to everything. *If I only knew then what I know now.* I never thought I'd say those words, but after 4 decades of life, I've come to realize I don't know as much as I thought I did. That little question no longer seems simple.

That's what led to another realization. The answer to that seemingly simple question couldn't be encapsulated in a label or a line I could add to my résumé. It required a deeper understanding of myself, a level of self-awareness that I had yet to achieve, and it wasn't going to land in my lap, either. I had to go get it, and it wasn't going to come from an external source, whether the media, my advisors, or even my family. It had to come from a place inside *me.*

I decided I needed an overhaul, and not just of my body this time. I wanted to develop a clearer frame of mind and also get back in tune with my spirituality. Reclaiming this essential part of me that has lain dormant for so long, combined with my passion for sculpting my body and eating properly, could, I felt, not just change me but *transform* me into the best possible version of myself.

My journey to become whole is what inspired this book. It's the natural successor to my first book, *LL Cool J's Platinum Workout,* because where *Platinum Workout* focused on the body, *P360* develops the total package.

Think of *P360* as a guide to strengthening the three pillars that make you who you are: your mind, your body, and your soul. It's taken me 40 years to recognize that all these elements are tied together—that you cannot be strong in body without being strong in mind and spirit. Now I'm ready to share these insights with you to help you develop into your most fully realized and powerful self. What's important to me is that you understand not just how to be fit and healthy but why you deserve to be fit and healthy. Once you've made that breakthrough, you'll find it easy to commit to a 360-degree package of mental, physical, and emotional health.

You will start the P360 program well before you set foot in the gym or eat a single serving of food from the nutrition plan. The very first step is changing the way you approach success by learning to manage your expectations and to think big—but start small.

Once I've put you in the right frame of mind to achieve your goals, it's time to get that body on par with your mind with the kind of simple but highly effective workout you've come to expect from me. To complete the P360, I've laid out a comprehensive diet designed to complement the Platinum Workout that not only shows you what to eat but also teaches you how the food you put in your body can dramatically affect your results in the gym.

But getting physically fit and committing yourself to a healthier lifestyle is just the tip of the iceberg. So many people seem to focus only on the body. They're only interested in the aesthetic. That's the equivalent of sitting down meal after meal and eating nothing but meat. No vegetables. No starches. No liquids. Not even dessert. Invariably, your body will begin to suffer because it's not getting everything it needs to function properly, and eventually you'll develop deficiencies so severe that even the benefits the meat offered in the first place will no longer do you any good. Now take that principle and apply it to your whole life. I firmly believe that the depth of your character and the extent of your patience are as important as the size of your biceps when it comes to being a complete, well-rounded individual.

For the last 8 years, I have been going through a physical transformation, a process I undertook for one simple reason: I was unhappy with the way I looked and it began to affect the way I felt. I vividly remember standing in front of the mirror and, for the first time in my life, being unhappy with what I saw. My body was changing, and not for the better. I began to feel insecure. I didn't feel like myself. The disappointment I felt when I looked in the mirror started a tidal wave of emotional resentment. Then it hit me. I didn't trust myself. I was no longer my own go-to guy. This wasn't the vision I had for myself.

So I did something about it. I vowed to lose 40 pounds, and with the help of the workout plan in *LL Cool J's Platinum Workout*, the first book in my self-improvement Platinum series, I lost 40 pounds.

The feeling of elation and satisfaction I experienced from the transformation of my body quickly made me realize that the benefits of being in great shape—and feeling good about the way I looked—directly affected how I felt physically and emotionally. It was my first glimpse into the interconnections between physical fitness, mental clarity, and spiritual wellness. And now with *Platinum 360*, I'll share with you what I've learned on my journey to becoming a complete, highly functioning person.

So who am I? For starters, I'm just like you. I've got dreams and goals; I've had triumphs and failures. I go through the same highs and lows that you do on a daily basis. And just like with you, if I don't work out and eat right, my body starts to suffer. I'm the kind of person who wants to get the maximum out of life. And in order to do that, I knew I had to change the person I saw in the mirror, physically, mentally, and spiritually, because that person, no matter what the reflection suggested, wasn't complete. He wasn't getting the most out of what life put in front of him.

So I did something about it. And with *Platinum 360*, you'll learn how you can, too.

I'm writing this book not simply to tell you what to do and how to do it but also to motivate you. Regardless of what I may look like on the cover of this book, there's always some area I think I can improve on, and I won't ever be completely done with this transformation process. So we're in it together. Think of me as your partner on this journey.

I am a driven person—if I do something, I want to succeed at it—and I know you do, too.

BEST DECISIONS I EVER MADE

CHANGE MY RAP NAME
I used to be known as J Ski, but when I went with LL Cool J, it felt like I took a creative leap. It ended up being timeless.

SIGNING WITH DEF JAM
I made my dream come true. It's what got everything started.

PURSUING ACTING
It was another way I could express myself creatively. It also meant I no longer had to rely on just music.

STARTING OTHER BUSINESSES OUTSIDE OF PERFORMING
I really began to see my true business potential. From there I became financially liberated.

GETTING IN SHAPE
Outside of the obvious health benefits, it changed my life 100 percent.

Nothing would make my journey more rewarding than to see you follow the road map I've laid out here so that you can look and feel better as a result.

Our bodies reflect our minds—when you feel good about yourself, inside and out, there's no challenge too great for you to face. You'll be back on your A-game, feeling positive about yourself and ready to go boldly after your dreams and live the life you've imagined with vigor, energy, and passion. By following the Platinum 360 program, you'll see a metamorphosis in your body that you never thought possible in such a short time. You'll look in the mirror and know that the trip was well worth it.

But let me be real with you. Total fitness—mind, body, and soul—can't be achieved in the short term. You can't put a month's worth of work into it and think you've finished the job. This is just the beginning of your passage to a better you. This isn't about going on a fad diet or running on the treadmill and hoping to shed a few extra pounds. This is committing to a better, healthier lifestyle.

THE PLATINUM 360 TEAM
I couldn't have done this alone. To reach my own goals, I put together the best team I could, which includes my trainer, Scooter Honig, and nutrition expert Jim Stoppani, who holds a doctorate in exercise physiology and studied the effects of diet on the body at Yale University School of Medicine. Between these two pros, I have the most up-to-date and proven strategies for keeping my body working at its highest level.

Scooter has been my fitness trainer for

9 years and worked with me to design the Platinum workouts that are responsible for my body's conditioning. (He also trains other celebrity clients and world-class athletes.)

When I want the best advice on nutrition plans to give me the energy I need to handle Scooter's workouts, I turn to Jim Stoppani. In addition to being an expert on exercise, Jim is a bodybuilder and nutrition planner for numerous celebrities, athletes, and fitness magazines. He knows his stuff on the science side of nutrition and also on how to implement it in the real world for real people.

So it made sense to have the guys that I rely on every day show you how to re-create your body. They helped me hone my personal philosophies and construct the Platinum programs. Luckily, though, you don't need to hire a squad of your own experts to get the same results. I have done all the hard work for you. All you have to do now is follow the plan that I lay out in this book.

LET'S GET THIS THING STARTED

I'm a hopeful person. Hope has always played a significant role in my life. And here's what I hope for you: When you're finished with this book, you'll be ready to live life to your maximum potential. I hope—no, I know—that you will be all that you can be. Make no mistake—putting forth the kind of effort it takes to maximize your potential is not easy. Most people decide to take the easy way out. Most people decide against putting in the work. But by reading this book, you've already taken the first step.

I'm not promising that it will be easy. You can't get something for nothing, and you can't improve your mind, body, and spirit without sacrifice. You have to suffer a little to get there. But wouldn't you rather suffer the pain of discipline as you strive to be successful than the pain of regret because you didn't go for your dreams? Discipline weighs ounces, but regret weighs tons.

My personal evolution is ongoing, and I know I am better today than I was yesterday. I'm on a continuous journey to discover who I am, and I am using that knowledge to become a better person. Do I know more today than I did the day before? Did I dig deeper within myself? Simply, how did I improve? I never stop examining the way I live.

I've dedicated my life to self-improvement. I've committed my life to excellence. I'm driven by the idea of maximizing my output and reaching *my* potential. I decided long ago that only things that will help me reach that end will be allowed in my circle.

The book in your hands is a primer for revealing a better you, a guide to finding out who you really are and becoming the person you always knew you could be. Prepare to fulfill *your* potential. You want to get better, don't you? Of course! Why else would you be holding this book?

So time to turn up the houselights and get started. The path to a better, healthier, and ultimately more fulfilling life starts *now*. I'll be with you every step of the way, but ultimately, it's up to you. It's your body. Your mind. Your soul. There's only one thing left to ask yourself.

Who are you?

PART ONE

LL COOL J'S
PLATINUM 360 PLAN
FOR SUCCESS

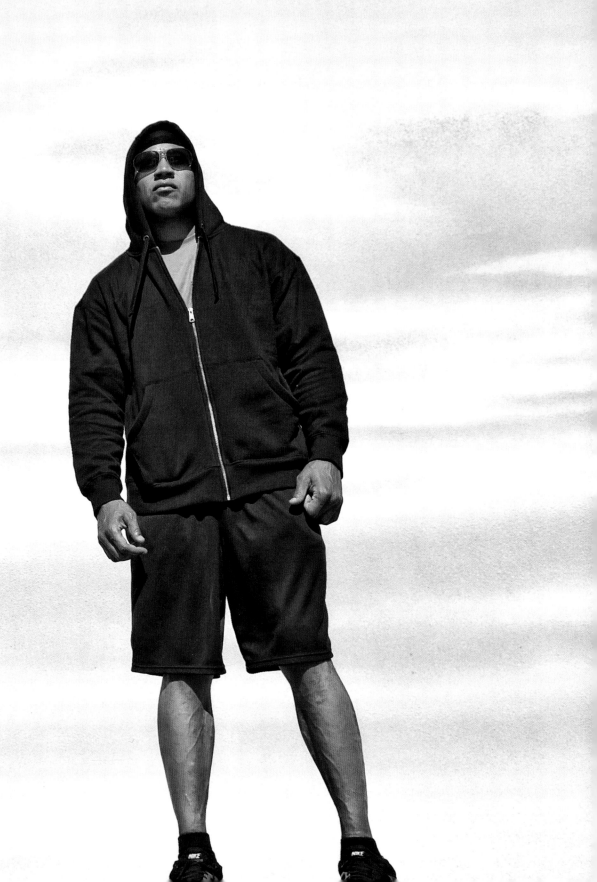

PREPARING YOUR MIND FOR SUCCESS

A fit, sharp mind is the foundation on which every major accomplishment is built. When you are mentally fit, you turn problems into opportunities. You are more likely to maximize the relationships you're in and less likely to succumb to depression, anxiety, and stress once you realize that your future is up to you.

You will find it easier to manage your life and thrive on new challenges instead of feeling burdened by them.

The first step is to create and maintain a positive outlook. Envision your future while you work to make it a reality.

If you can see it, you can be it. Envision a life for yourself, then set out to achieve that dream. No need to broadcast it to the world. Just go do it.

In many cases it will take a lot of your energy to keep yourself motivated. No one's going to throw a parade for you. Oftentimes you'll be your only cheerleader. When the going gets tough, remember that determination is one of your most valuable resources. It will put you in the proper frame of mind to deal with setbacks and the inevitable bumps in the road. In other words, when the elevator is broken, you will turn around and take the steps. It could very well decide whether you reach your

personal mountaintop or settle for someone else's version of success—or even worse, failure.

Along the way, you may discover the need to adapt, change, understand, and accept different viewpoints and approaches. Don't worry. That's just self-improvement at work. Be open to new things, then decide what's right for you.

Think of your life as a company and yourself as the CEO. Even though the CEO is the one calling the shots and making the decisions, he or she doesn't run the company alone. A good CEO seeks feedback and advice every day before deciding what's best for the company. Learn from the people around you. See if they can help you improve your process. Family, friends, colleagues, classmates, and community can be an indispensable part of your efforts to achieve your goals. Success doesn't happen in a vacuum; it's often a communal effort.

Much as the goal of physical fitness is to achieve a stronger, healthier body, the purpose of this section is to strengthen your mind. You'll learn how to do this through positive reinforcement that will build your confidence, which in turn will make you a force to be reckoned with. Exercise by applying these principles, tips, and rules to your everyday life. Throughout this section, I give examples from my life that helped me develop the level of mental fitness I have today. Many of the rules or principles I lay out have already been taught to you at some stage of your life. The problem is that you may have disregarded them as "just something parents say" or just plain old common sense and are therefore not applying them correctly to your daily life. Remember, common sense isn't common.

Sometimes all it takes is a little reinforcement together with a little proof that the principles actually work. Want proof? Look no further than yours truly. These are the very same thoughts and watchwords that I've used my entire life to shape my personal philosophies and to strengthen and exercise my mind. They're the key to all of my accomplishments. Different people might take a little something different from each of these principles. Find what works best in your life and go with it.

Life is full of things to deal with: relationships, career, family, and everything that goes along with them. It can get complicated. You're never going to have all the answers. If you did, you wouldn't need this book. But if you have a strong and sound mind, your definition of success will be that much clearer and that much closer to achieving.

No matter how you define success, there are essential steps to take before you begin the process of becoming the person you've always envisioned. It won't happen in a day, and your progress won't be a straight line. Expect to fail, but don't accept it. Thomas Edison failed thousands of times in his life. So did Albert Einstein. But you're not trying to invent something that will change the course of history, you're just trying to find the best possible you. I'll be glad I had a hand in helping to motivate you.

But for right now, stay focused on the present. Your new life starts now. This is your guide. You'll be in the gym soon enough to focus on the physical, but for the moment you need a checkup from the neck up. Trust me, when you get yourself in the proper frame of mind, with success in your scope, you'll have set the stage for achieving your goals both in and out of the gym.

Consider the time you devote to strengthening and sharpening your mind prep time for real-world situations. When you are prepared, there isn't a single obstacle that can stop you from traveling your path to success, even if you have to take a few detours on the way. The time you devote to preparation will pay dividends on the back end. This is your new life, and you owe it to yourself to make the most of it.

Let's get started.

CHAPTER 1
DARE TO BE GREAT

I've always been someone who made things happen for myself, maybe because I was an only child. I had to create things on my own, and I was probably a little impatient, too. I just never wanted to wait. I was the kid who didn't wait for his parents to put the hammock together. They came home and it was already put together. When I was 8 years old and playing peewee football, I realized my mother had forgotten to put my uniform in the wash. No way was I going to the game in a dirty uniform. I wasn't quite sure how to use the washing machine, but I figured it out. I got to the game in a uniform that was still wet, but at least I had done it myself.

Look, there are three types of people: those who understand on their own, those who understand when they're told, and those who never understand. I always understood on my own, but self-starting is difficult. Master it and you'll give yourself a head start to your dreams.

So be proactive. Don't wait for someone to tell you to begin. Don't wait for life to throw you a curve or deal you a bad hand before you decide to take charge. Do it now.

Have a vision. When you have a clear vision of your goal, it's easier to take the first step toward it. If you don't have a vision or a plan, there's no reason to take that step.

SET YOUR GOALS AND STICK TO THEM

A writer named Edward De Bono wrote "A man without a goal is like a cork floating on the ocean." He doesn't control his own destiny. You're at the mercy of the ocean, and where you end up is up to the tide. Goals are the building blocks of your overall life plan. If you're the kind of person who orchestrates the day around whoever knocks on the door at any given moment, then you don't have a plan. That's being rudderless. I can't remember the last time I didn't have a strategy for the day and specific goals to conquer, even if I got just one step closer. That's how I operate every day of my life.

CULTIVATE YOUR IMAGINATION

The whole idea that man is the architect of his own fortune is something I subscribe to. If you can dream it, you can be it. Imagination is a powerful tool as well as a gift. If you want something, you have to see it in your mind before it can happen. The great thing is that these dreams don't have deadlines. A lot of people get the sense that if they didn't envision a specific career when they were kids it's too late by the time they're adults. Doesn't work like that, but thinking like a child helps. There's nothing more pure and honest than a child's imagination. Children can dream up anything. They don't understand the concept of I Can't as it relates to dreaming. They are free of all that nasty, toxic drama that adults carry and can easily envision the places in life they want to visit. If a kid can brush aside No and I Can't, so

can you. I call it having the right type of innocence, something that's pure and joyful and passionate and comes from a place of love. Innocence doesn't equal naïveté but, rather, purity. When you find that within yourself, you'll see that imagination just bursting out of you and its manifestations taking place in your life.

MAXIMIZE YOUR POTENTIAL, not someone else's. If there's one thing life has taught me it is that comparisons will kill you. Imagine you have a 5-gallon bucket. Someone else may have a 10-gallon bucket. Don't get caught up in the size of anyone else's bucket. Fill your own. You never know, when he fills his 10-gallon bucket, he may not be strong enough to carry it. So don't worry about the size of your bucket. Just fill the one you have.

WHEN YOU LOVE WHAT YOU DO, IT'S NOT A JOB

Do what you love; you'll be better at it. It sounds pretty simple, but you'd be surprised how many people don't get this one right away. Bill Gates would not have pioneered the software industry if he didn't have an absolute fervor for personal computing. Kobe Bryant, Denzel Washington, and anyone you can think of who is at the top of his field wouldn't be there if not for the love they have for what they do. That's not to say love alone will vault you to the top of whatever career path you choose. But that love will get you through the rough patches. It will keep you from throwing in the towel when you think the weight is too heavy.

Listen, I love being fit even though getting there is tough sometimes. I wouldn't be in the shape I am in if I didn't enjoy working out. Yeah, sometimes it's a pain and I don't always feel like dragging myself to the gym, but it's what I'm passionate about. When you find something you love to do that much, make it your life's work; you'll be a lot happier than if you convince yourself to make a living doing something that your heart isn't in. Love what you do and your life will be better for the experience.

PLAY YOUR ROLE

Find value in whatever you do. In the body of mankind, some people are toes and others are elbows. Some are lips, while still others are kneecaps. Whatever you are, make sure you do it well. If you're an ear, make sure you can hear. If you're an eye, make sure you can see. If you're a hand, know how to grab. If you're a leg, you'd better be able to hold the body up. No role is insignificant. If you're a toe but you're broken, the entire body will limp. Play your position. Don't be concerned with rank. Make sure you're in the role that maximizes your capabilities.

LIMITATIONS ARE A FIGMENT OF YOUR IMAGINATION

Only when you identify your limits can you exceed them. I say you should look at limits simply as a measure of how far you have come, a benchmark that, once attained, will quickly be surpassed when you set a new goal. If your ultimate goal is to bench-press 200 pounds, find out what you can realistically (and safely) do right now, and set your first goal at 10 pounds more than that. Once you master that level, reset your goal, and repeat the process until you achieve your goal of bench-pressing 200 pounds. Who knows, you may find that the goal you once considered unattainable is not only attainable, but can be surpassed through determined and focused effort.

Limitations come from many kinds of different sources. They can come from our own minds due to a lack of self-confidence, or they can be thrust upon us by others. If everybody in your neighborhood thinks you're going to grow up to be a failure, you could start to doubt yourself. That's a limitation. It may be as simple as a lack of money or transportation or the proper tools to get to where you want to be. Sometimes limitations can be both physical and mental. Whatever they might be, identify them. Acknowledge your limitations and move past them.

NOVEL IDEA: BE YOURSELF

Do you know anyone who has tried to model his life on someone else, be it a celebrity, a family member—whoever? They say imitation is the sincerest form of flattery. I say imitation is the number one killer of individualism. Be yourself. It's who you were meant to be. But people often see possibilities in others and only limitations in themselves. If you see a man driving a nice car, you may want that car, but you have no idea about what kind of hard work, struggle, and sacrifice he may have had to go through to enable him to have a car like that. Sallust, a Roman historian, once said, "If they envy my distinction let them also envy my toils." If you never look beyond the persona, image, or public façades of anyone who seems to have the things you aspire to, it's easy to feel like everybody's life is better than yours. You're thinking that all you have is struggles, setbacks, and one obstacle after another. Well, believe me, the guy with the fancy car has obstacles of his own. So instead of wishing you were in the car, you could be tackling the obstacles that stand between you and that car by being true to your vision. Be yourself; everyone else is already taken.

FACE YOUR FEARS

One of my favorite quotes is from Martin Luther King Jr., who said: "If you know it's the right thing to do but you're afraid, do it anyway." A lot of people will stay in a dead-end job or refuse to venture outside their comfort zone simply due to fear. Sometimes life requires you to step away from what's familiar to you, from what's safe, in order to go after what you truly desire. Imagine a guy working at a comfortable job that pays a good salary. You might look at him and think he has it made, even though beneath the surface he's unhappy, uninspired, and downright frustrated because he's not doing something he's truly passionate about. He thinks about following his passion to another career all the time but is afraid to attempt the transition because he's been in his comfort zone for so long. My advice is simple: Go do it. Now.

Sometimes you have to put your gloves on. Stand up and face your fears, or they will defeat you. The key is don't make things bigger than they really are. Imagine you are standing in front of a 2-foot-wide chasm that's just a foot deep. You could jump over it with no more thought than you'd take stepping off a curb. Now imagine that same chasm 2 feet wide but 1,000 feet deep. The thought of jumping over it makes your body tense up. Sweat starts to bead on your forehead. All of a sudden, you're psyching yourself out despite the fact that it requires no more physical skill or exertion than the first jump. When I decided I wanted to pursue acting, I had to be willing to bare my soul. It wasn't an easy thing to do. I was worried that it would affect my music. I knew

PESSIMISTS DON'T MAKE HISTORY

Don't be a naysayer. All that accomplishes is telling people you're so shortsighted, you couldn't find the solution if it was right in front of your face or, even worse, that you're unwilling to look for one. There's a Chinese proverb that observes those who say it can't be done should not interrupt the person doing it. Don't be the guy who says man wasn't meant to fly then looks surprised to see the Wright brothers soaring over his head. In the 1800s, a politician proposed closing the patent office because he thought that everything that could be invented already existed—not exactly a visionary. What if Thomas Edison's colleague constantly told him the lightbulb would never work? You'd probably own a lot of candles.

that I was going to have to step outside of the image that I had cultivated in the music industry and be a different guy. I knew that I might be called on to play a character that wasn't cool or to be vulnerable, and that was a scary thing. But I moved past it. I didn't let the fear close off my options or limit my dreams. Don't let the fear dominate you. I often find that when you overcome your fear, you'll look back and wonder what you were so afraid of. Facing your fear will set you free.

BE DETERMINED, STAY HUNGRY

Determination is your biggest asset. It's a mind-set that enables you to tell the world you will not be denied. When you approach a task or goal without a determined attitude, every little obstacle that falls in your path will throw you off track. Without determination, you run the risk of becoming a serial quitter, someone who's always beginning things and quitting instead of following through because you're not applying your will. Approach *everything* you do with determination.

I know it's easy to say, but it's a lot more difficult to live by this rule in your daily life. What has always fueled my determination was my burning desire to accomplish my goals. Being determined was instilled in me from a young age by my mother and grandmother. *If a task is once begun, never leave it till it's done; be the labor big or small, do it well or not at all.* This was the mantra I heard every day, and I still consider those words to live by.

Not everybody has those built-in raging fires, but that's okay; stick-to-itiveness can be a learned behavior. You can change the way you think about dealing with obstacles. Instead of fearing obstacles, you'll come to embrace them. See them as a challenge, a wall between you and your goal, but one you can scale with the right tools and effort.

MOST INFLUENTIAL PEOPLE IN MY LIFE

SILVER FOX—OLD-SCHOOL HIP-HOP ARTIST/MEMBER OF FANTASY THREE
When I was a young rapper, he helped me put the finishing touches on my rap style.

RICK RUBIN—RECORD EXECUTIVE/PRODUCER
Gave me my first break. That simple.

RUSSELL SIMMONS—FOUNDER, DEF JAM
He never infringed on my creative style, and he taught me the power of being me.

QUINCY JONES—MULTI-GRAMMY-WINNING MUSIC PRODUCER
The man taught me a lot about class and generosity.

SEAN "DIDDY" COMBS—HIP-HIP MOGUL
In his own way, he showed me that I didn't have to be just an artist.

PERSEVERE—BUT PERSEVERE CORRECTLY

Now you might be thinking we already covered this, but in my mind, determination and perseverance are two different things, separate but definitely equal. I see perseverance as having more in common with endurance. They work hand in hand, but determination precedes perseverance. You can't persevere before you become determined. In order to get the most out of your perseverance to keep yourself on the right track, you've got to know when and where to persevere because you could spend 10 years persevering on a path that leads directly into a brick wall, and what good does that do? Be selective in your perseverance, but always be determined.

ONE LAST POINT ABOUT DETERMINATION

The difference between impossible and possible is your determination. Just ask Knicks guard Nate Robinson. There's a person with no shortage of determination. At 5-foot-8, he not only made it to the top of his profession as a basketball player, but he also won the Slam Dunk Contest. Being short is an obvious disadvantage when it comes to the NBA. Throughout his life, Robinson was constantly told he wasn't tall enough to succeed at the elite level of basketball, and he became determined to prove people wrong. But you don't need a 44-inch vertical leap to persuade naysayers with the power of your determination. Whether you're a 45-year-old mother of three who wants to return to school to get her degree or a community leader who dreams of opening a youth center in his old neighborhood, it all comes down to determination. Your determination will fuel your success. It's a simple yet extremely powerful tool.

TREAT "NO" LIKE DIRT—BRUSH IT OFF

Let's face it, hearing *no* is a fact of everyday life. Whether you're an artist, a screenwriter, or a salesman, people are quick to tell you no. People are trained and conditioned to say no. It's the safe thing to do. It saves them from risking themselves no matter how great your idea might be. The word *no* is designed to discourage you. Don't let it. Turn it around and make it work for you. *No* should make you stronger. Every time you hear it, become more resilient, more focused, more determined. Rethink your strategy, but don't lose sight of your goal. One time I interviewed for a special effects–driven movie that I really wanted to do, but

the director just wasn't feeling me. That's his prerogative. It happens. Did I get discouraged? No, I kept pushing forward. Soon after, I got the role in *Deep Blue Sea*, which ended up being a terrific experience. *No* is only an obstacle if you let it be. And remember, one *yes* can erase a thousand noes.

WHEN THE CHIPS ARE DOWN, PICK 'EM UP

When a seed is planted, it's deep below the surface of the earth, underneath the soil, where it's dark and cold and wet. There are bugs and earthworms everywhere. Even when the seed begins to sprout, it's surrounded by darkness and its situation seems hopeless. Then, all of a sudden, BOOM! It breaks through the surface and sees the sun, and the flower is born. The point is, when the chips are down and it seems the darkest, success could be really close.

But sometimes it doesn't seem like the seed is going to sprout. Sometimes you just miss the writing on the wall and failures happen. But that's where it gets interesting. Even if you don't reach a certain goal when you want to, you never truly fail. There's always another chance, another way, another day. Okay, so you didn't hit the target this time. Just keep it moving. Don't be the one who digs 900 feet and gives up. What if the next person behind you digs 3 more feet and strikes gold? You would not feel platinum.

THE BLAME GAME

You want to know the easiest way to lose track of your destiny and put power in other people's hands? Blame them for your problems. When you blame others, you give up your power to effect change. When you point the finger at others instead of looking in the mirror, you're letting yourself off the hook. If every failure or disappointment in your life is someone else's fault, there's no need

YOU WERE ONCE THE BIG MAN on campus—

get over It. Live out of your imagination, not your history. You may have thought you were the greatest thing that ever happened to the world when you were in high school. You were a whiz with the ladies, had a great fastball, and threw the best parties. All your friends and coworkers know about this because you remind them every chance you get. But at some point, you have to take off that class ring. Sometimes the biggest obstacles in our path to success are the memories in the rearview mirror. Don't cling so tightly to the past; you'll find you're just holding faded memories after a while. Go out and be great today. At the very least, you'll have some new stories to tell. Don't let your past hold your future hostage.

for you to improve, right? If you get a less than glowing work evaluation and blame your boss, you're skirting responsibility. And don't point a finger at your teacher if you get a bad grade. Are you taking into account the fact that you didn't study or pay attention in class or that participation was 20 percent of your grade? And who decided not to do the extra-credit assignments? Whose fault is it

that you don't know the causes of the Civil War, your teacher's or the fact that you didn't do the required reading? If it were the teacher's fault, there would be no reason to study harder. If you blame others, you give up the power to change. The power to succeed goes right along with it.

HANG ON TO THAT BRAIN—YOU'LL NEED IT

Taking risks and trying new things is a big key to happiness and success. But be smart about it. As Richard Dawkins wrote, don't be so open-minded that your brains drop out. You've heard the saying "I'll try anything once." Many people say it for the sake of fitting in or out of the need to impress those around them. But don't let that need force you into a situation that you could regret for the rest of your life. You wouldn't play Russian roulette once, would you? Not unless the thing you want to fit into is a coffin.

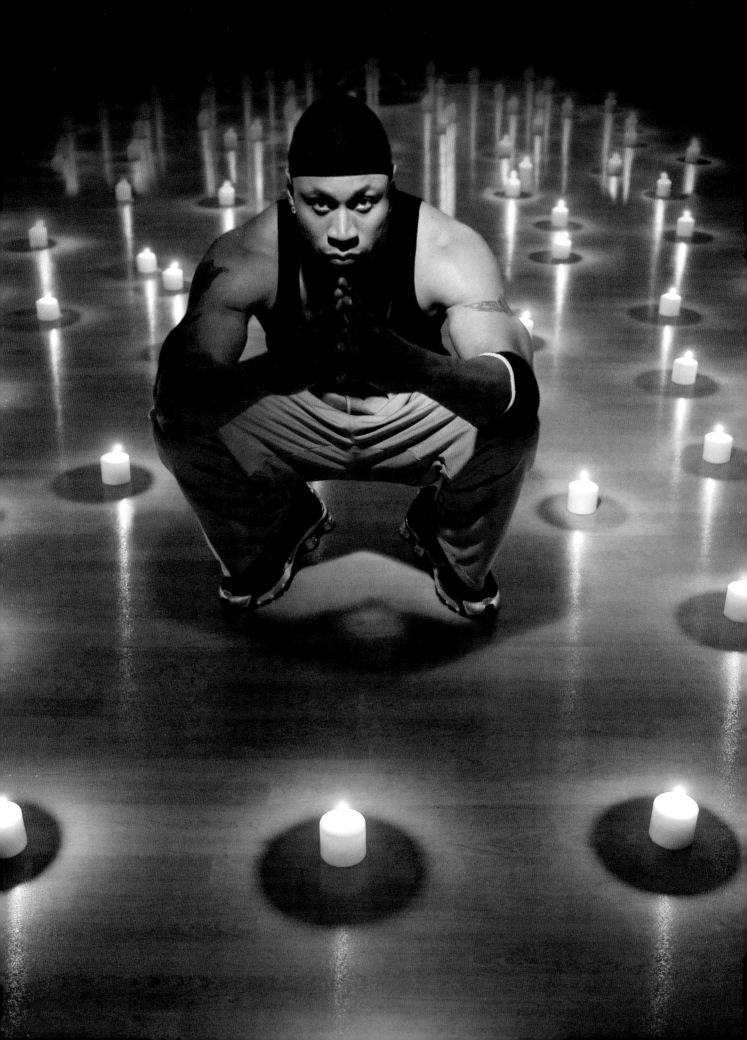

CHAPTER 2
YOU CAN'T DO IT ALONE

Having a family really changed my outlook on how I approach life. When you're single and without a family, you tend to live for yourself. When you take on the role of family man (or woman), your priorities change. Now you have to take care of people other than yourself. That doesn't mean your needs come last; in fact, the opposite is true. I realized that the only way I could take care of my family was to take care of myself. I call it the flight attendant theory. Put on your oxygen mask before helping others. Having a family made me want to get every phase of my life in order because I was responsible *to* other people as well as *for* them.

HELP ME, HELP YOU

I will take care of me for you if you will take care of you for me. Imagine this: You and your friend have decided to go into business together. It's agreed that you're going to handle the business end and your partner will take on product development. You begin to line up potential investors and sketch out a solid marketing plan. One day, you check in on your partner's progress only to find he's way behind on developing the products your company plans to sell. His plans are a mess and his research is incoherent. He's just plain disorganized.

Now the investors are ready to see the wonderful proposal and product demonstration you and you partner have put together—only you don't have anything to show them because your partner hasn't done the front-end work. In other words, he hasn't taken care of himself for you. If he had, his presentation would be in order. When I do my part to get myself ready, it will benefit you. When you do your part, it will benefit me. Together we prosper. This adage extends way beyond business. The same principles can be applied to friendship. If we take care of ourselves for each other, our friendship can survive anything.

TILL DEATH DO US COMPROMISE

The beauty of marriage is that you have someone with whom to share your dreams, a person with whom you can face and conquer all of life's obstacles. But marriage is not a fairy tale. It's not as simple as meeting someone and falling in love. You have to work at it. You have to know when to compromise. If I want to go to LA but she wants to be in Miami, we have to find a third location that will satisfy both of us. The end goal is to settle on something that makes both of you happy. That's making it work.

There are many moving parts within a marriage, but every successful marriage is built on these three pillars: trust, love, and communication. Call it the TLC of marriage. Trust is the foundation without which no healthy marriage can survive. Love is as important as the air we breathe. It fills in all the gaps. Imagine your marriage as a flower;

GETTING EVEN

If you must get even with somebody, get even with those who have helped you (John E. Southard). Don't waste your energy trying to get even with people who have slighted you. Vindictiveness is not a positive quality. Success is the best revenge. Ultimately, taking the high road is the sign of a confident, humble person. If you put aside all of the slights, petty jealousies, backbiting, and poisonous behavior and instead reciprocate the good done to you, it's a much more empowering way to live.

love is the water and sunlight it needs to grow. Communication is what enables two people to work things out. If you think you'll never have anything to work out, then don't get married. You will. Hearing each other's side in a dispute and establishing an open dialogue ensures that miscommunication won't turn a little thing into a big blowup or a big thing into a divorce court proceeding. When you think about it, these principles can be applied to any healthy relationship.

IT DOESN'T COST A THING TO PAY ATTENTION

One of the greatest gifts you can give anyone is the gift of your attention. It's like Miracle-Gro for your soul. Have you heard a little kid who's about to jump in a pool or do a cartwheel yell out, "Mommy, look at me"? Children naturally seek attention. When they receive it, it tells them someone cares what they are doing and that they are loved. Attention, like food, water, and shelter, is a basic human need. We can't thrive or grow without it. A lot of troubled teens who get into mischief or act up in class are reacting to the lack of attention they've had throughout their lives. People want to be heard, and that never really leaves you as you get older, although you may learn to deal with it better. Attention makes us feel worthwhile. Remember that even in the most straightforward situations. Take a conversation, for example. It's not just an opportunity for you to get your opinion across to the person in front of you; it's extremely important that you listen to what the other person has to say as well. If you were in a room full of people, and the president of the United States walked in and talked with you for 30 seconds, that would likely have a huge impact on you. All he did was give you a few moments of attention, and you could take that with you forever. Who knows what you'd be inspired to do after that? Best of all, you don't need to be the president to have that kind of effect on somebody. Just try it. It doesn't cost anything to pay attention. All you have to do is stop, look, and listen.

GANDHI WAS RIGHT

If you don't like what's happening in your community, do something about it. Let it start with you. As Gandhi said, become the change you want to see. Don't wait for it to change. Change it.

The community you live in, whether you realize it or not, shapes who you are as a person and vice versa. And while you may move away one day or live in several different places over the course of your life, you should always leave your community a better place than you found it. Some people who come into your life are like scaffolding that exists temporarily on the side of a building. Whenever you see scaffolding, you know someone is working to improve the building's structure or appearance. When the scaffolding is removed, you can see the benefits of those efforts.

In life, each person serves as the scaffolding for someone else's life. You impact those around you every day. When you part ways with that person, his or her life should be better for the experience. Treat your neighbors with respect and they will reciprocate. If you look at them with a distrustful eye, they will return the favor. And then you're not living in a community but, rather, with a collection of people in close proximity who don't support one another. Eventually, the scaffolding crumbles to the ground and the building is left worse than before.

PEOPLE I ADMIRE

BARACK OBAMA
He accomplished what people thought was impossible.

MICHAEL JORDAN
His work ethic was no joke.

BOB JOHNSON
He founded BET and became America's first African-American billionaire by navigating the labyrinth of business.

DENZEL WASHINGTON
Even after Sidney Poitier, Denzel opened doors for African-American actors and let them know they could be leading men.

MY GRANDPARENTS
They showed me the importance of hard work, determination, and loyalty in life.

HOW MANY OF US HAVE REAL FRIENDS?

Friends are people you share love, joy, and good energy with. Being there for another person is a cornerstone of friendship. To have friends, you have to be friendly yourself. When someone really needs you, you have to be there. A friend should help you achieve your goals and dreams and help you get to a place in your life that you couldn't have reached alone. Say you want to start a business, kick a drug problem, or walk away from a bad relationship. A true friend will join or support you in any one of those endeavors unconditionally. As you go through life, you'll have mountains to climb, some big and some small, and—let's face it—some of them you won't be able to scale alone. I'd be willing to bet the people who help you along the way will be friends for life.

If someone in your life isn't willing to give that kind of support, then that person is probably more of an associate or acquaintance than a true friend. Friends are the ones who build you up, not those who come around after you've made it. But friendship is a two-way street. The trust, love, and support you're seeking must be reciprocated. One-way friendships usually don't last too long. Imagine a kid who aspires to go to college. Everything he dreams about achieving is within his reach if he gets that college degree. It's the night before his SATs. He needs a great score to get into the school of his choice—and his buddy is throwing a party to end all parties. When the birthday boy finds out that his college-bound buddy can't attend because he needs to get his rest, he lays a guilt trip on him. He feels his bookworm friend is letting him down. So who's really being a bad friend? To me, it's the guy who's throwing the party. He's getting in the way of his buddy's dream, and all he has to offer is one night of partying. That's not true friendship. True friendship is helping your friends achieve their goals.

WHAT THE EYE SEES

One day a man woke up to find his ax missing. He went outside and saw his neighbor's son walk by. To the man's eye, everything about the boy said he had stolen the ax: the way he walked, the way he moved, the surreptitious way he glanced over at him. There was no doubt in the man's mind that the boy was guilty.

Then, later that night, the man found the ax in his own garage, where it had fallen behind some other tools. He felt like a fool for having blamed the neighbor's son when the boy had nothing to do with the missing ax. The next morning he saw the neighbor's son, and nothing about him suggested an ax thief. The boy was no different, but today he didn't seem at all guilty.

But friendship is not simply about being friendly. If I just sat there and listened to you complain about your life for hours on end, I don't think I'd be much of a friend. A real friend wouldn't allow you to do that. A real friend would offer something more constructive than a sympathetic ear: a way to help you correct whatever it is that's giving you trouble or holding you back. That's helping you become something better than you already are. Remember the scaffolding. A true friend is one who helps you build something. A real friend is not only scaffolding but part of the foundation.

Faith, Love, Respect, and the Little Things, Too

OVERCOME THE CRITICS

Do you know how many people don't try new things out of fear of criticism? It prevents them from going after their dreams every day. Stops them cold. Holds them back. Chains them down. Some people become so concerned about what others might say, they'd rather not hear them say anything at all. They convince themselves that the best way to avoid criticism is not to make an effort that can be judged in the first place. This fear of criticism can be debilitating. Imagine if everyone had that mentality. What if a farmer felt inadequate about his crops and gave up? We would starve. If everyone thought like that, we wouldn't have great music or artists or athletes or engineers or doctors or teachers. What if Michael Jackson had been afraid of having people judge his music? We would have been deprived of an incredible body of work. Fear of criticism is an incredibly powerful deterrent. Conquer it and your options will be limitless.

PURE OF HEART

Nothing good can be achieved without purity of heart. A good heart trumps someone else's bad intentions any day. When you can see the good in others, people are drawn to you. But there is a distinction between a good heart and a foolish one. The latter will get you

nowhere. A foolish heart trusts others blindly even while being deceived.

Remember when Lucy would hold the football for Charlie Brown to kick and then pull it away at the last second? Charlie would kick and miss and land flat on his back every time, without fail. Of course, Lucy would swear up and down that she'd hold the ball in place the next time, and Charlie would line up to kick the ball again. Then he would inevitably wind up on his back. That's a foolish heart. He trusted even while he was being deceived and made a fool. Unfortunately, there will always be plenty of people waiting to take advantage of your naïveté. Don't be Charlie Brown.

GET YOUR SELF-ESTEEM IN CHECK

Positive self-esteem is one of the major building blocks of success and happiness. Love yourself. Respect yourself. Know that you are someone who deserves success. Without good self-esteem, you are susceptible to having others shape your view of yourself. There are those in your path who would try to take advantage of this, but if you have a healthy sense of self-esteem, they'll just be wasting their breath. Think of a basketball player who's out on the court talking trash. He's trying to discourage his opponent through words. Always remember that words are just words. Confidence in yourself and your abilities is like a suit of armor. You'll be protected from those who try to lower your opinion of yourself. Most of the time self-esteem is tied to the way you look—we'll get to your physical well-being in the next chapter—but understand that your goal is not to live up to someone else's standards. You simply have to be the best you that *you* can be. Nothing more.

OVERCOME DOUBT

Much like fear of criticism, doubt can stop you cold. The difference is that doubt comes from within. Doubt is digging up the seeds before they grow. Doubt is the opposite of faith. When you doubt, you are expressing your belief that something *won't* work and that you don't believe in yourself. Doubt is something we all face. Those nagging questions about our own abilities creep up and follow us around as we go through life. The key is being ready and able to deflect doubt before it stops you from reaching your ultimate goals. Believe me, no one ever accomplished anything after succumbing to doubt.

HAVE CHARACTER, DON'T BE ONE

How do you judge character? By a person's good deeds? By how nice someone is to others? Sometimes what a person refuses to do is equally revealing. When a high school basketball star is offered $10,000 to accept a college scholarship and turns it down because he knows it's against the rules and doesn't want to jeopardize his amateur status, that is an example of character. When you show a multi-

tude of positive moral attributes—loyalty, courage, honesty—you quickly develop a reputation for being of sound character. I think it ultimately boils down to doing the right thing.

KEEP THE FAITH

The Bible teaches us that faith is the substance of things hoped for and the evidence of things not seen. Believing in something is part of human nature. Faith is belief plus action. If you need to believe, keep taking action. I've always believed faith is contagious. Surround yourself with those who are faithful, and you'll feel your own faith strengthening.

Have character. Don't be one. Being a character is being someone no one takes seriously—somebody who's developed a reputation that he doesn't stand for anything. Character is standing for something. Remember what Malcolm X said: "When you don't stand for something, you will fall for anything."

RESPECT: EARN IT AND GIVE IT

Getting and receiving respect has always been tremendously important to me. It sets the table for basic human interaction. It keeps the order and the peace. Seeing how my grandfather conducted himself taught me how important respect is in defining your relationships with everyone around you. The way he treated others, his family, and himself made a lasting impression on me. He fixed his own cars, cashed his checks, put the money on the table, and was always home for supper. He never failed to let his wife know she was everything, his rock. Watching my mother—a single mother—work so hard and always retain her dignity gave me respect for people who have to walk that path. When you understand how important respect is, you'll know how important it is to give it. You can tell a lot about people by how they relate to people they don't think they need. I believe in giving a janitor the same amount of respect I would a CEO. They can choose to lose my respect, but in the beginning, I treat everyone equally. Some people will give you a rope so you can hang yourself. I'll give you a rope so you can climb.

GOOD IS GOOD, BUT GREAT IS BETTER

I live my life by one motto: Good is the enemy of great. Don't settle for good. If you settle for good, you've already failed. Listen, good is fine, but don't be afraid to give up the good to get the great. Greatness is the only thing really worth striving for. Say you have a solid job as a mail carrier. Pays decent bucks, puts food on the table, and the work is enjoyable because it provides fresh air and exercise. But in the back of your mind, as you go from house to house dropping off letters and catalogs, you dream about going back to school to get that degree in business administration so you can open up your own business. Of course, that would require taking fewer hours at your job—or working toward your degree after hours and sacrificing sleep time, which in turn might end up costing you your job. You've checked your finances carefully, and it looks like you can get by until you complete your degree, but you would likely have to sacrifice a certain level of comfort for a few years. That trip you were planning to Vegas this summer? Forget about it. Your employer might even replace you or not allow you to work a part-time

schedule. Either way, to chase that degree— and possibly a better life—you'll have to take some risks and step out of your comfort zone. You could fail, but you could become greater than you've ever imagined.

SHOW ME SOME LOVE

There is no stronger force in the universe than love. Always operate from a place of love. Let that be your core responsibility. Where others are afraid to carry the load, you have to pick up the slack. Love doesn't weigh a thing, but hate is a burden too strong for most to bear. It's like having a bee in your shirt stinging you over and over. When you're held down by hate, it's a terrible way to live. Love always overcomes hate. Many people think if they live their lives guided by love, they'll be seen as a doormat. Love is not weakness. Love is strength. Love will never be defeated. When you have love in your life, the psychological and emotional benefits are manifold. You're excited to face the day. You have a bounce in your step. You're far less likely to become depressed or lie around all day in a funk. Love is like oxygen for the soul. It keeps you breathing. Love creates understanding. It's why people with obvious differences can get along. But love isn't self-sustaining. It doesn't just automatically keep running. It needs to be nurtured. You have to work at love because love is often tested. The stronger your love is, the more it takes to break it. To get love and keep love, you have to give it. The more you give, the more you'll get in return. Love fends off depression and sadness, so when you give love, you are literally improving someone's health. That's reason enough to show the love. Just remember Charlie Brown (wink).

KEEP YOUR PASSION—SOMETIMES IT'S ALL YOU'VE GOT

Passion can propel anyone from the most humble beginnings to the highest peak. I'm a perfect example. I'm from a hard-scrabble, brown-bag-over-the-40-ounce, two-tokes-and-pass kind of neighborhood. I had to travel a long way to get to where I am today, but I always believed I could do *anything*. Because my mom always told me, "Todd, you can do anything you put your mind to," she kindled my faith and passion. To this day, I still believe I can accomplish anything I put my mind to. If I wanted to pilot the space shuttle, I could get it done. But it's not just me. Anyone can accomplish what they choose. You have to believe it. You have to breathe it. It has to be part of your spirit. It has to be part of your essence. The courage to fulfill your vision comes from passion not position. Passion will get you to the position you ultimately desire.

CHECK YOUR REP

A reputation is like your calling card. It's how people know you, so you should take care of it because you only get one. But here's the rub— don't obsess over it. After all, reputation, much like beauty, is in the eye of the beholder. It's very subjective. Do all you can do to the best of your ability. Know at the end of the day that you gave everything you had. If you're sincere in your actions and pure of heart, you'll be fine, and your reputation will speak for itself.

PLACES THAT INSPIRE ME

PARIS, FRANCE
There's just so much beauty there it's humbling.

CÔTE D'IVOIRE, AFRICA
I went there and felt like I was home. They crowned me a king, and it humbled me.

ITALY
The architecture is just breathtaking. That area has given birth to so many great minds, I can't help but be inspired.

HARLEM
All the guys I hung out with had that go-get-it mentality and were always on the grind. They proved to me you could get what you wanted if you worked hard enough.

CHAPTER 3
ADAPT, ADJUST, AND ABOVE ALL, NEVER STOP LEARNING

There's something I call having the confidence to be humble. True humility is the absence of ego. Everyone has an ego and a natural inclination to protect it. But if it grows too big, it will only get in the way. No one wants to work with someone who has an oversized ego. It's a surefire way to turn off friends, bosses, potential clients, and people you're meeting for the first time. That's your ego getting in the way. When you're confident enough to be humble, you don't need your ego to validate who you are.

When you find comfort in being who you are, you don't have to put on any airs. You don't want to be a pretender. That never accomplishes anything. Those who put on airs are not experiencing the type of success they envisioned for themselves; if they were, they wouldn't have the need to posture. They're hiding something, and as long as that's the case, they'll never achieve what they really want. It may seem to you that others have a lot, but it's not what they truly want. And maybe it's not as much as it appears to be. Have the confidence to be humble.

BETTER BE SHO'

It's not what you don't know that gets you into trouble; it's the things you know for sure . . . but aren't so. Always be certain, but make sure you're certain about the right thing. If you and a friend are caught in a burning building and you say, "I know for an absolute fact that this is the key to the emergency exit," you will save the day. But if you get to the door and the key doesn't work, things are going to get mighty hot for the both of you. There are some mistakes you don't get to make twice. One of the biggest mistakes you can make is to be certain about the wrong thing. If you're playing matchmaker for your best friend, be certain you know the character of the person you're setting her up with. If you're giving directions and think you know a shortcut, make sure it's really the shortest route before you swear by it. No one likes bad information. The fact that you really, really thought it was true doesn't make it any less wrong. It won't make you look any less foolish, and it won't make them forgive you more quickly. Here's a bonus tip: Even when you're certain you know the "right" answer, be cool about it. Keep your ego in check. You'll maintain your credibility in the long run.

THINKING IT DOESN'T MEAN YOU HAVE TO SAY IT

If you don't have anything positive to say, then it's better to say nothing at all. Everybody has been told a variation on this theme at one time or another. It's one of the first things a parent teaches a child. Fundamentally, this time-honored adage points to one thing: Be kind. Perhaps there is someone in your life you sim-

READ, LEARN, GROW
Jim Rohn, a motivational speaker, once said, "Miss a meal if you have to, but don't miss a book." One of the best ways to self-improvement is reading the collected knowledge of those who have come before you. Pick up a book. It's like going to a gym for your mind.

ply don't get along with. You've tried, but at the end of the day, you just plain don't like them. Do yourself and everyone around you a favor: Keep your feelings to yourself. Don't contribute to the poison. I deal with entertainment types for a living, and not everyone I meet becomes my favorite person. Colleagues often ask me about someone I'm not so fond of. Sometimes it's better to just smile and move on. The kindest word is the unkind word unsaid.

THE ONE PRISON THAT CAN'T HOLD YOU

You don't have to be convicted of a crime to go to prison. I'm not talking about the brick-and-mortar Shawshank variety. I'm talking about a prison of the mind. Many people are held captive by their own belief that they can't achieve success. They don't think they're good enough and that happiness and success are only meant for others. It's a terrible thing to lock yourself up. It can affect a kid who doesn't have the confidence to go out for the football team or some-

EVERY HOUR COUNTS

If you're upset with how much you earn, here's a suggestion: Work harder. Ultimately, you don't get paid for the hour, you get paid for the value you bring to the hour, as Jim Rohn says. That's why different people earn different hourly wages. So bring more value to your hours. Your boss may not compensate you at the end of this week or the next, but you're paving the way to a promotion by making yourself more valuable to the company. Even if your boss does not recognize your value, another employer or potential partner will. The easiest way to get paid more is to do a great job and more than you're paid for.

body from an impoverished neighborhood who thinks he's destined to live a life of poverty because that's all he's ever known. Defeating thoughts like these are what get you booked into that prison of the mind. Negative attitudes have locked people up for centuries. The good news is that it doesn't have to be a life sentence. With a change of attitude, you could be free tomorrow. When life has you handcuffed, the key to freedom is your thoughts. Only the right thoughts can unlock your mind. And your mind determines how you will live your life. More often than not, the key is right in your own pocket. All you have to do is reach for it.

ENVY KILLS

"Why him and not me?" "Why is she getting a promotion when I've been stuck in the same job for 3 years?" "Why does my teammate have a better jump shot than I do?" Any of these questions sound familiar? They should if you're human. We all experience envy at some point in our lives. It's part of the human condition. We look at what our neighbor has and wonder why we are without. We always covet what we don't have. Envy will only distract you from reaching your goals. How can you achieve what you want when you're so busy looking at what your next-door neighbor has in his garage? Most likely you won't. When you look at someone else's success, you can either let it magnify your own perceived shortcomings or use it as inspiration. If you're an intern and one of your peers is on track for a corner office, use it as motivation to work on your jump shot. Don't waste time with envy when motivation is all around you.

CAUTION: POISONOUS VIBES AHEAD

Why so bitter? When you're angry with someone and you let it fester, that person has taken control of your happiness, whether you know it or not. If a coworker makes a disparaging remark about you, handle it and move on. Don't let it weigh you down. When you harbor resentment, there's a poisonous vibe seeping into your everyday life. Do you think you'll ever be happy sniffing poison all day? Take a moment and set down that baggage. It's giving you a hump in your back. The day you decide to let go of the resentment, anger, and bitterness you've been carrying around is the day you can truly take responsibility for your own emotional well-being. When you take responsibility, you grow up. You accept that your happiness and your success are up to you. Here's the bonus: Now you've empowered yourself to make changes in your life. One of the sweetest forms of revenge is to be happy, healthy, and successful.

READ THE WRITING ON THE WALL—IT COULD BE ADDRESSED TO YOU

Every day of your life, you encounter signs pointing you in the right direction. Some of them are right in front of your face while others you might not notice as easily. Often these signs—both obvious and subtle—are indicators that you're not exactly taking care of business. They can be simple. You keep missing the bus to work because you're always running late. That's a sign that you need to get up earlier or go to bed at a decent hour. Maybe you need to streamline your morning routine. Only you know for sure. Either way, when you find yourself running down the street with your coffee in your hand and your briefcase flying open, it's probably a sign you need to pay attention to. Sometimes the stakes are much higher. Imagine a teenager in an impoverished neighborhood who thinks selling drugs is an easy way to get money. His cousin was arrested and given a 20-year sentence and his best friend was killed in a drug shootout, but he thinks that can't happen to him. Those are some pretty big signs to miss. They're telling him it's time to make a positive life change or risk the same fate as the rest of his crew. Don't let the inability to learn from other people's mistakes doom you to make the same ones.

WHAT YOU SEE DEPENDS ON HOW YOU SEE THINGS
Two guys are sailing across the ocean and come to an uninhabited island. They dock their boat and set off to explore the new land. The trip has been arduous, and they realize they could be lost for days. After a while, they come upon a barefoot indigenous population. One of the travelers frowns while the other smiles. One sees a backward people out of touch with the rest of the world. The other sees a new customer base for his nascent shoe company. A pessimist sees the difficulty in every opportunity; an optimist sees the opportunity in every difficulty. When you see opportunity in every situation, you increase your chance for success. An optimist sees a gateway. A pessimist can only see a closed door. Same situation, different view.

OBJECTS IN MOTION TEND TO BE MORE FORTUNATE

If you want a fortune, you have to be fortunate. And fortune favors the bold. That means you're infinitely more likely to experience good fortune if you get out there and try as opposed to sitting around on your couch all day. If you're one of those people who think fortune is just going to knock on your door, my only advice for you is to get a comfortable couch and a lifetime's worth of supplies, because that's how long you'll be waiting.

GET BETTER— IT'S THE ONLY OPTION

Time spent wishing something was easier is time wasted. The things worth going after will be at the end of very difficult roads. That's the way life works. Get used to it. Don't sit around and wish things were easier. Get better. I have

BIG MISTAKES I LEARNED FROM

SELLING OWNERSHIP OF DEF JAM TOO EARLY

I felt I needed the money and sold my ownership in Def Jam way too early. If I had been patient, my stake would have been worth much more.

PICKING WRONG MANAGERS

At the beginning of my career, I was in the habit of elevating people who weren't elevating me and didn't have the ability to do so.

CHOOSING FRIENDS FOR THE WRONG REASON

I used to surround myself with people who were just fun to have around. Ultimately, I realized they were no good for me.

NOT FULLY UNDERSTANDING THE CONSEQUENCES OF MY BUSINESS DECISIONS

Early in my career, I was all about signing the contract. But I often didn't even understand my rights or power to renegotiate a better deal.

a news flash: If you want to be a stock market whiz, there's no failsafe manual telling you exactly what to buy and sell. Doesn't exist. People have a tendency to want to make the obstacle smaller rather than make themselves bigger. But you are the only part of that equation that you control.

SOMETIMES YOUR SHIP WILL SINK—JUST MAKE SURE YOU'RE NOT ON IT

Colin Powell often says, "Don't let your ego get too close to your position, so that if your position gets shot down, your ego doesn't go with it." It's one of my favorite quotes, and I try to live by it daily. To me it means to stand firmly for something but be flexible. Be able to adapt if your position isn't well received. When you're an artist like I am and make a living in such a volatile and subjective field as the music business, you would do well to take that advice to heart. Take my last album, for example, *Exit 13*. The single "Baby" did pretty well, but the album didn't meet my expectations in terms of sales and commercial success. Now, I could give you a lecture on the problems with the music industry, but they're beside the point. The fact of the matter is that the album didn't resonate with my fans the way I wanted it to. The point is I didn't allow my ego to get so caught up in the success of the album that if it didn't become a smash, I'd be sitting around feeling miserable. I couldn't write a book about becoming the best you can be if that was the way I thought. So your project fails. Be tough. Move on. Thomas Edison failed 10,000 times before he invented the lightbulb. What if George Foreman had never come back after being defeated by Muhammad Ali in Zaire? None of us would be flipping turkey burgers on a Foreman grill. Would Barack Obama have changed the world if he had given up politics after losing the race for the Illinois state senate in 2003? Don't let your ego fool you into being embarrassed if something you've done doesn't become an international phenomenon. In other words, don't get too close to your position. You don't have to go down with the ship. The next idea you have will serve as your life raft or, better yet, the mega yacht of your dreams. Never forget, every failure is a brick in the castle of success.

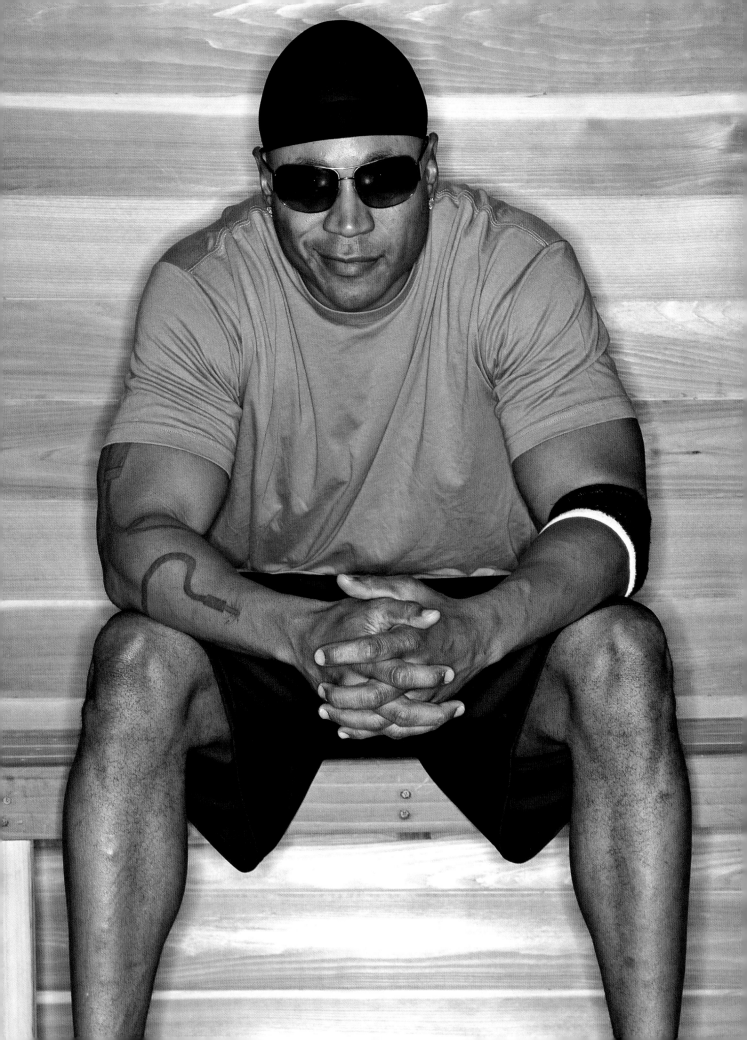

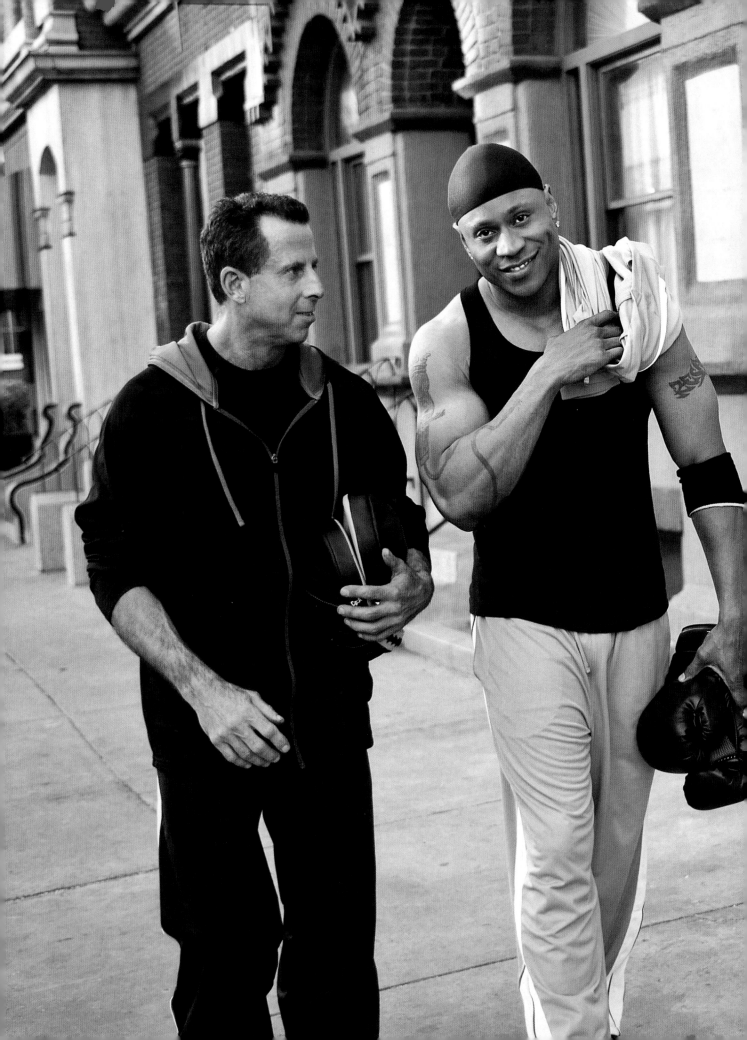

PART TWO

THE PLATINUM 360
FITNESS PLAN

Wow, talk about lessons to last a lifetime. I know what you're thinking: That was a lot to take in. So don't try to. America wasn't built in a day. You won't be, either. Step back. Decompress. The previous section was designed for you to take what you want when you need it and apply it to your life whenever applicable, since there is no specific order to revamping your mental and spiritual outlook.

But now we're going to step into the portion of the P360 plan that's a little more rigid and structured. When you hit the gym to continue your 360-degree transformation, I'm going to put you on a tighter path.

Your 8-week transformation will begin with a 2-week program geared toward men and women who are relatively new to working out with weights and cardio. But that doesn't mean that if you've been going to the gym for a few months (or even a few years), you won't benefit, too. Sometimes, when you're not operating at an optimum level over time, it's good to dial back and, well, start over. Your body may need to simply relearn the basics—heck, you may have been pushing it too hard (and in the wrong direction) for too long and just reached a stage of burnout.

In Weeks 3 and 4, you take one step toward a slightly more advanced regimen, dividing all your main body part exercises into two workouts instead of tackling a head-to-toe session. Whole-body work-outs have their place, especially for begin-ners, and even the most elite-level athletes can benefit from sometimes revisiting this technique. It's a test of strength and will to be able to train all your main muscle groups in the span of one 30-to-60-minute session. However, for the most part, the best results for physique enhancement arise when you can devote more attention and energy to individual parts of your body. By splitting it over more than 1 day, you have more energy and enthusiasm to devote to the body as a whole.

That's why you'll take the split concept even further in Weeks 5 and 6, splitting your muscle groups over three distinct workouts. Now things will start to get more intense, but in a good way, as pushing your limits is the only way you'll make the gains you really want. You should notice some interesting developments at this point in the form of a bit more muscle tone, more strength to handle more weight on your exercises, and an ability to bounce back from a workout faster with less muscle soreness. These are all signs that your workouts are working for you.

Just when you think you're getting your bearings, the fourth phase will arrive, and you'll be introduced to a stunningly effective workout intensifier: drop sets. We'll tell you more about how they're done in the explanation for that week, but as a preview, they go a little something like this: You do as many reps as you can handle with a heavy weight, then—without resting to even catch your breath—you drop some of that weight and continue the set. It'll build a fierce burn in your muscles like you've never felt before. Learn to like the burn; it's definitely your friend. The phrase "No pain, no gain" may be overused, but it was born from the truth. Those of you who test yourselves and don't just stop when workouts become uncomfortable or too hard will be the ones boasting the most dramatic, awe-inspiring results at the end.

Speaking of a test, Scooter's Advanced Program will feel like one! In Chapter 5, we introduce you to a dynamic form of training called plyometrics. It may sound like an odd word, but if you ever took gym class in grade school, you've done plyo-like exercises. It's simply things like jumping up and down or side to side or performing a pushup where you get off the ground. Performing dynamic, explosive plyometric movements and cardio activities like jumping rope between standard weight-training sets exposes your muscles and your whole body to a unique new stimulus.

Why is that important? To develop, the body needs a steady dose of change, or muscle confusion as it is commonly known. For instance, say you take any one of the phases in this workout and just do it in perpetuity. Week after week, month after month, you do that same program over and over and over again. All of a sudden, a workout that works wonders when placed within an overall structure like the one we provide will become useless. Why? The human body is extremely adaptable, and over time, it will adjust and be able to take on that routine—it loses any prompting to re-create itself.

In Chapter 5, you'll also find a cheat sheet for quick 30-minute workouts. Use these streamlined routines when time doesn't allow for a full-on gym session or when you want to focus on one particular part of your body.

I'm glad you made the choice to get in shape. This plan will get you there. It is constructed on proven principles that have helped millions shape an all-new physique for themselves. But here's a secret we have to share: There are lots of workouts in the world that will all work to a degree and that help you make a decided difference in your appearance. However, absolutely none of them can work forever. Over time, you have to expand your knowledge of weight and cardio training and be able to tweak your training sessions. Trust us, if you're committed, you'll get there. Over the next 8 weeks, you'll learn a lot about working out in general and about yourself in particular. And best of all, you'll be transformed, mind, body, and spirit.

So are you ready for 8 challenging, exciting, and rewarding weeks? Let's go!

CHAPTER 4

THE PLATINUM 8-WEEK WORKOUT PROGRAM

While the Mind section had no concrete time restraints, I've laid out a workout plan that will have you well on your way to a new body in just 8 weeks. On the following pages, I provide a complete training plan that both men and women can use. It's simple enough that someone just starting to work out can follow it without a hitch, yet challenging enough that even an experienced fitness buff can generate results. Just be sure to start with weights that allow you to complete the indicated reps comfortably at first, and add weight as you progress.

Keep in mind that there are no shortcuts to a great body—okay, so that's the bad news. But the good news is that, since there are no real "secrets," anyone can improve their physical fitness, gain newfound muscle tone, and really transform themselves. It's all about hard work, consistency, and a well-built plan. After finishing the Mind section, hopefully you've honed that motivation muscle to the point where nothing can stand in your way. Good, I thought so. Now here's the plan.

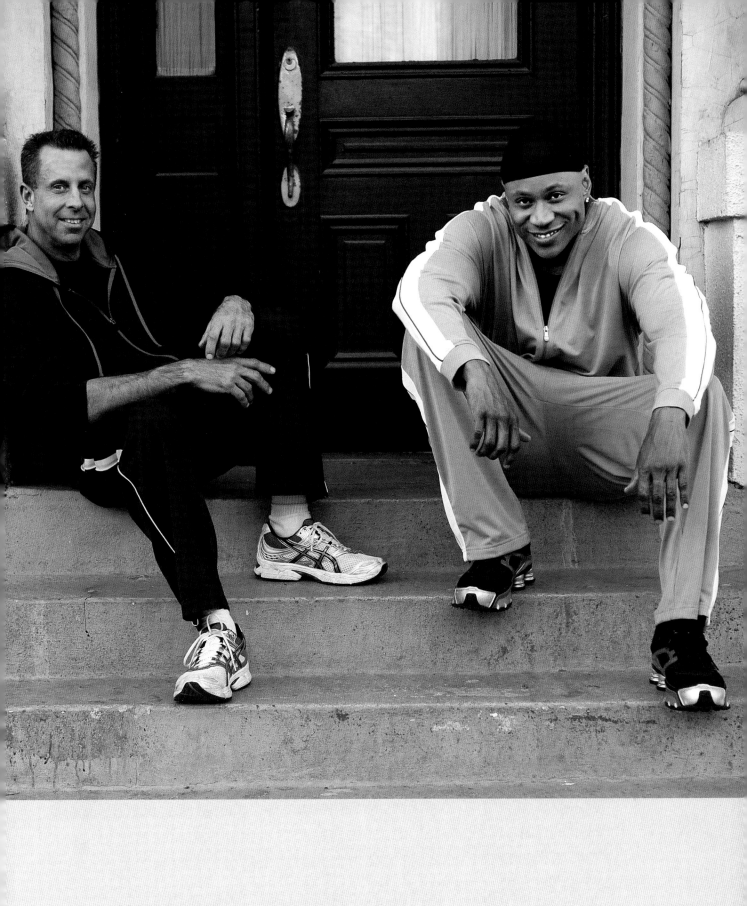

PHASE 1:
Weeks 1 and 2
Start Strong

In the first 2 weeks, you'll go to the gym and focus only on machine-based exercises, which are great for beginners or those returning to training after a long layoff. Why? Because they take away the element of balance—the machine safely balances the weight for you and fixes your path of motion so you can focus solely on the muscles doing the work.

In this phase, there is only one workout. The session includes exercises for your entire body, with 12 to 15 reps per set. Choose a resistance that challenges you, meaning it's a little tough to complete that 15th rep, but for now do not take sets to muscle failure, where you absolutely can't perform another rep with good form. That will come soon enough.

In this phase, you'll alternate machine workouts with steady-state cardio workouts, just taking it at a slow and easy pace, for 20 minutes. You can choose to run, jog, bike, or make use of the various cardio machines at the gym.

To those of you out there who are true beginners—that is, weight training for the first time—you may want to repeat this first phase two times before moving on to Phase 2 of the program and beyond. It'll get you acclimated to lifting and prepare you for the hard but effective workouts to come. In other words, you have to get in shape to get in shape.

PHASE 1 TRAINING SPLIT

DAY	MODE
1	Machine only
2	Cardio—20 minutes
3	Machine only
4	Cardio—20 minutes
5	Machine only
6	Cardio—20 minutes
7	Rest

Weeks 1 and 2 Workout

Perform this machine-only workout three times per week on nonconsecutive days (such as Monday, Wednesday, and Friday), alternating with cardio workouts.

Exercise	Sets	Reps
Leg Press	2	12–15
Leg Extension	2	12–15
Lying Leg Curl	2	12–15
Lat Pulldown	2	12–15
Machine Chest Press	2	12–15
Machine Row	2	12–15
Overhead Machine Press	2	12–15
Machine Preacher Curl	2	12–15
Cable Pressdown	2	12–15
Standing Calf Raise	2	12–15
Crunch	2	12–15

Rest 1 minute between sets; does not include warmup sets.

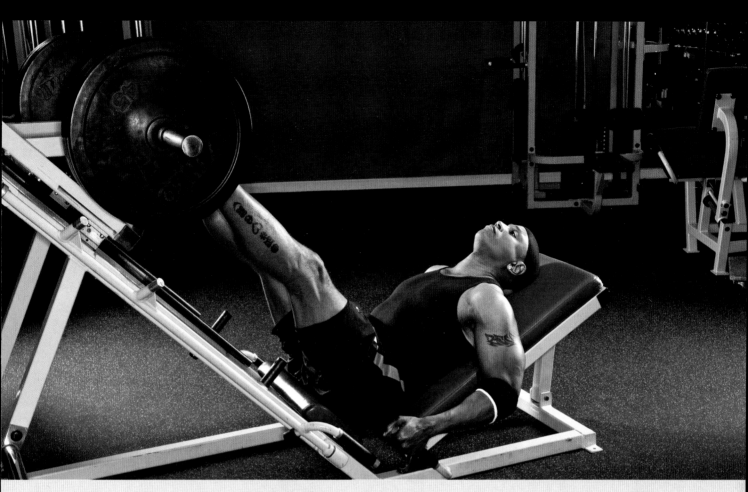

Leg Press: Sit squarely in the leg press machine and place your feet on the sled, shoulder-width apart. With your chest up and lower back pressed into the back support, carefully unlock the weight from the safeties. Bend your knees to lower the weight, stopping before your glutes lift off the pad. Hold for a brief count, then extend your knees to press the weight up, stopping just short of locking out your legs. Squeeze your thighs and glutes hard at the top before continuing the rep.

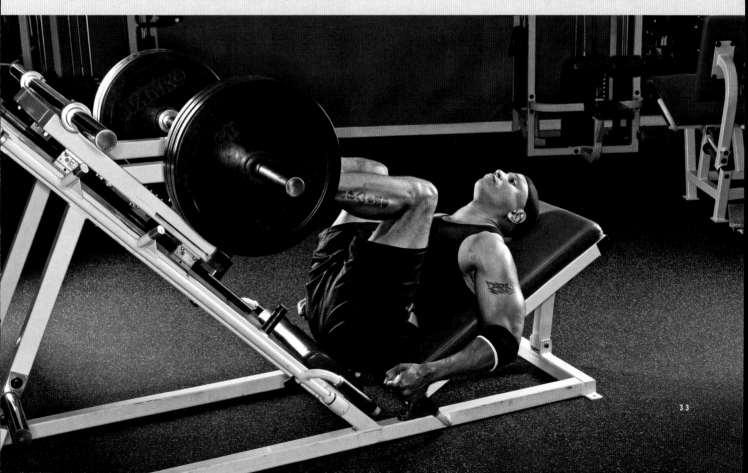

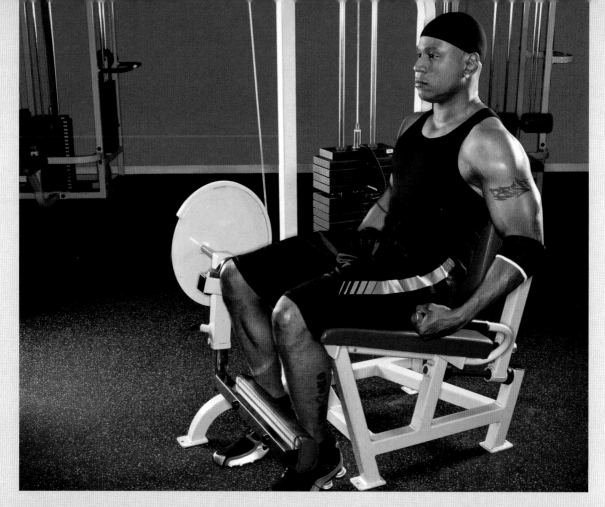

Leg Extension: Adjust the seat for your body frame, then sit squarely in the machine, hooking your feet under the pads. Keep your head straight and hold the handles for stability. With your feet pointed forward, extend your knees while remaining seated flat on the machine. Squeeze your quads hard at the top, then slowly lower the weight until just short of the weight stack, touching down before starting the next rep.

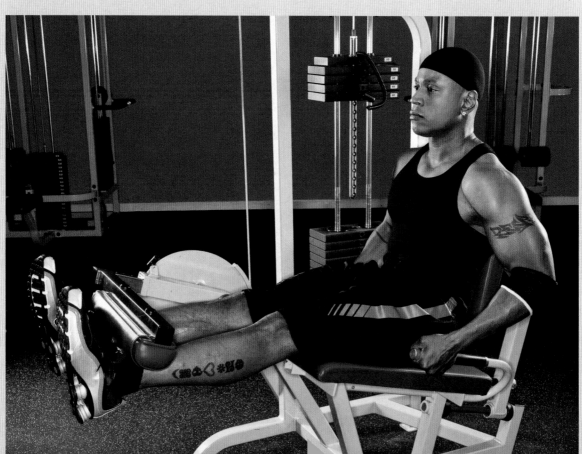

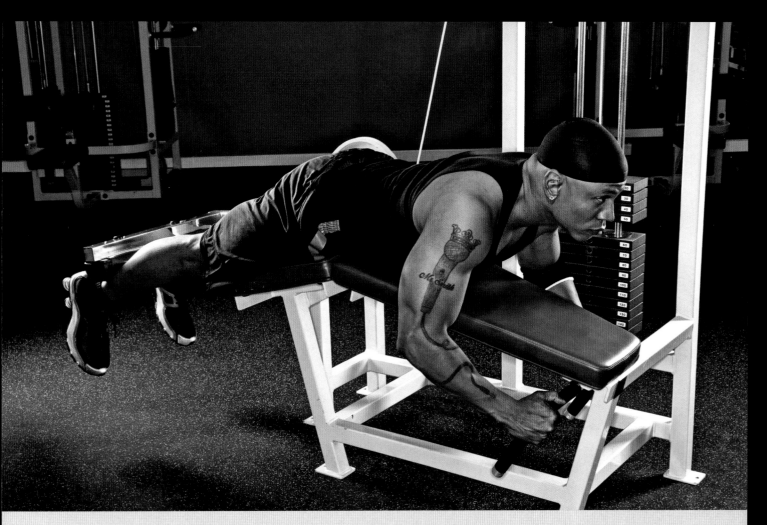

Lying Leg Curl: Lie facedown on a leg-curl machine and position your Achilles tendons below the padded lever, your knees just off the edge of the bench. Grasp the bench or handles for stability. Make sure your knees are slightly bent to protect them from overextension. Raise your feet toward your glutes in a strong but deliberate motion, squeezing your hamstrings at the top, then lower to the start position.

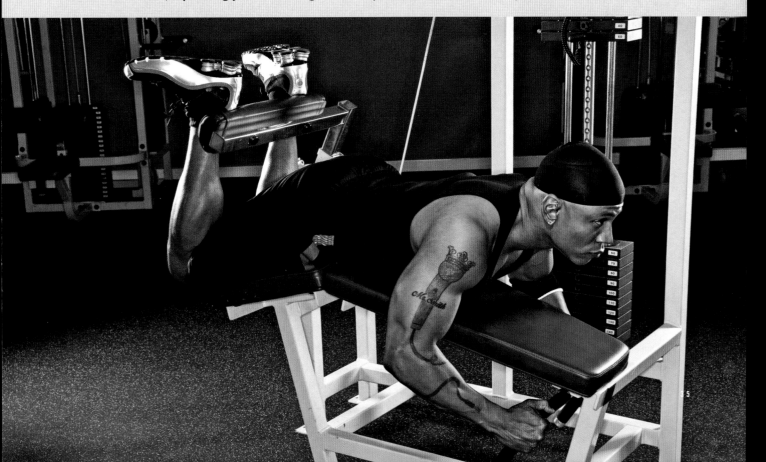

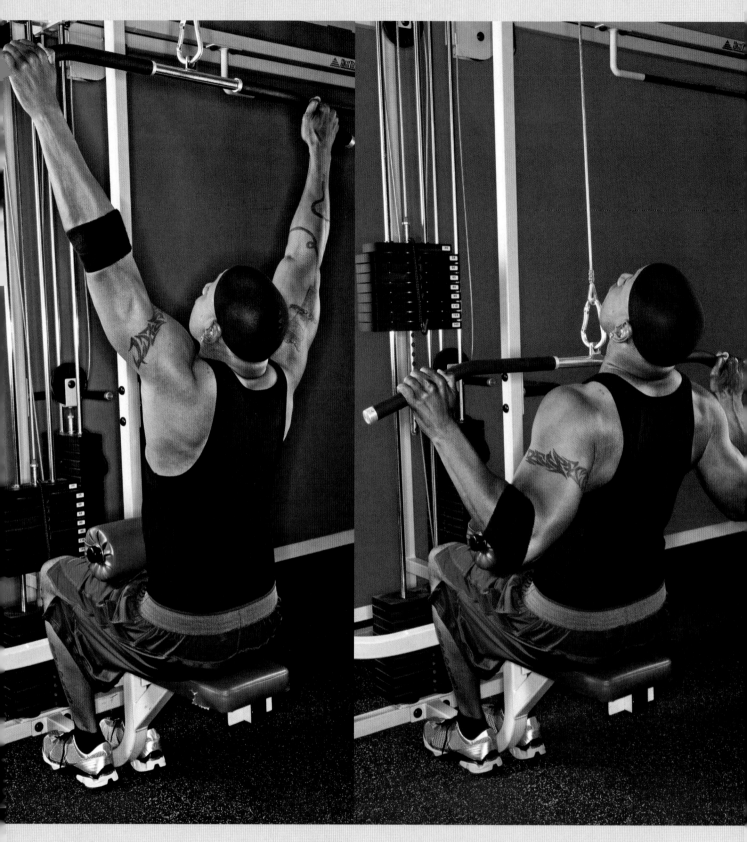

Lat Pulldown: Sit in a lat pulldown machine so the bar is slightly in front of your body. Adjust the pads so that your quads fit snugly over your thighs. Grasp the angled ends of the pulldown bar with a wide, overhand grip. Keep your abs tight and back slightly arched, with your feet flat on the floor. Squeeze your shoulder blades together and pull the bar down to your upper chest, keeping your elbows back and pointed out toward the sides in the same plane as your body. Squeeze and hold for a brief count before slowly allowing the bar to travel up along the same path.

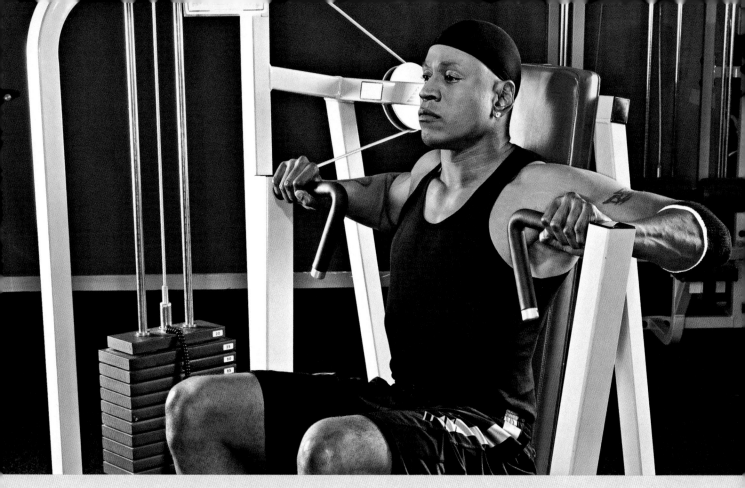

Machine Chest Press: Adjust the machine so your back rests comfortably against the pad and your feet are flat on the floor. The handles should be aligned right at or just below shoulder level when you sit down. Press the handles away from you until your arms are fully extended without locking out your elbows at the top. Slowly bring the handles back toward your chest without letting the weights touch the stack and repeat.

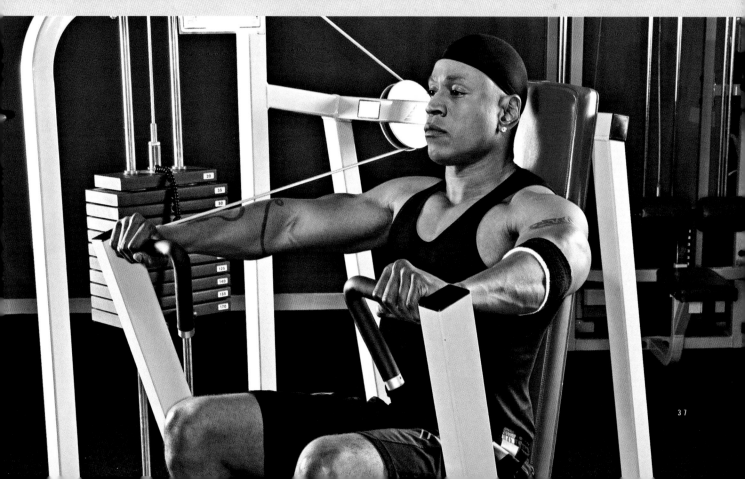

37

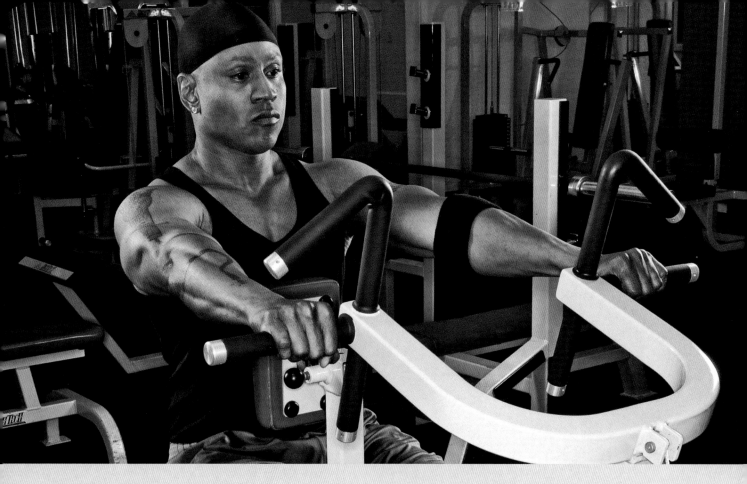

Machine Row: Sit in a selectorized row machine with your feet flat on the floor and your chest pressed against the pad. Grasp the handles with either a neutral or overhand grip and pull the handles toward you, squeezing your lats briefly. Return to the start position and repeat.

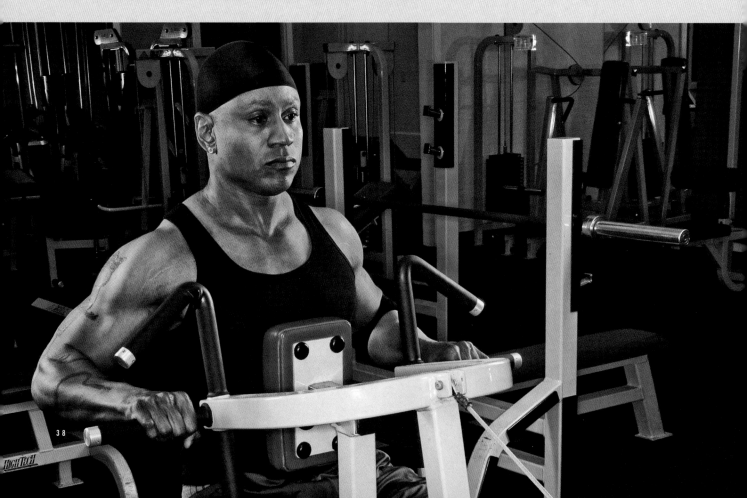

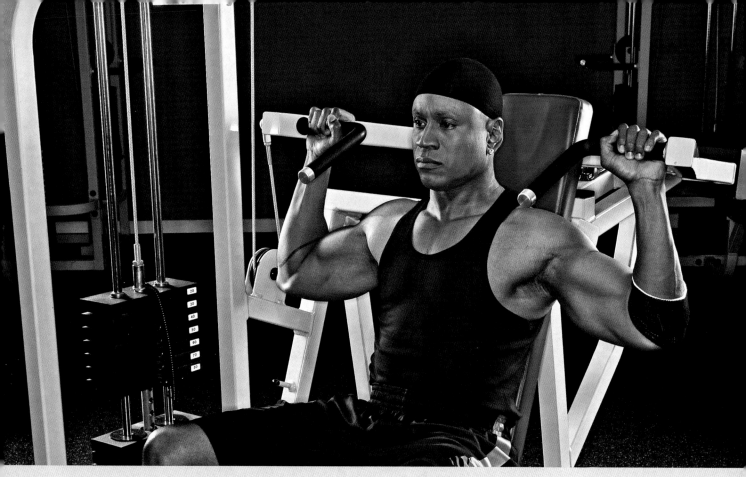

Overhead Machine Press: Adjust the machine so your back rests comfortably against the pad and your feet are flat on the floor. Grasp the handles and press them upward until your arms are fully extended without locking your elbows at the top. Slowly bring the handles back toward the plane of your delts without letting the weights touch the stack and repeat.

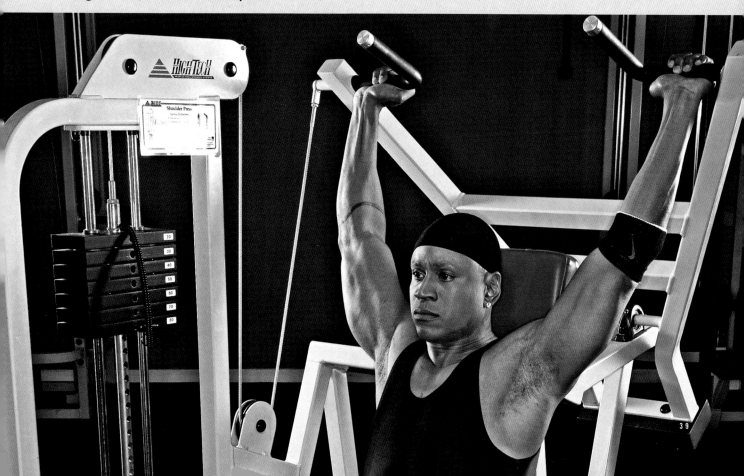

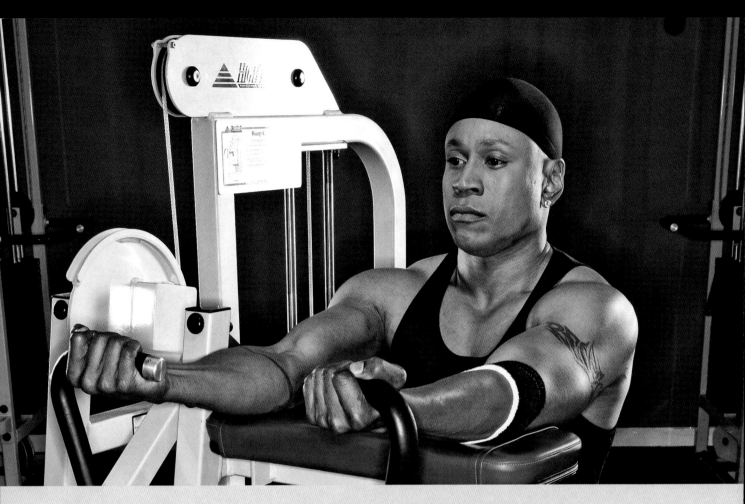

Machine Preacher Curl: Place your upper arms snugly against the pad and grasp the handles. Curl as high as you can, keeping your elbows on the pad, then lower to a point just before the weight stack touches down and begin the next rep.

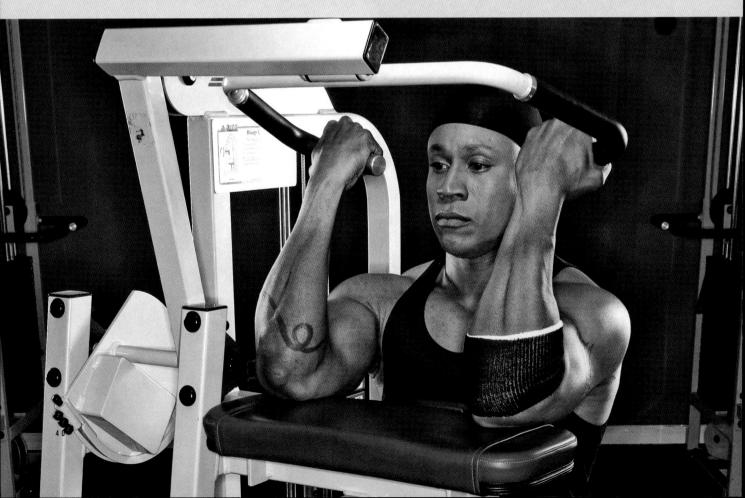

40

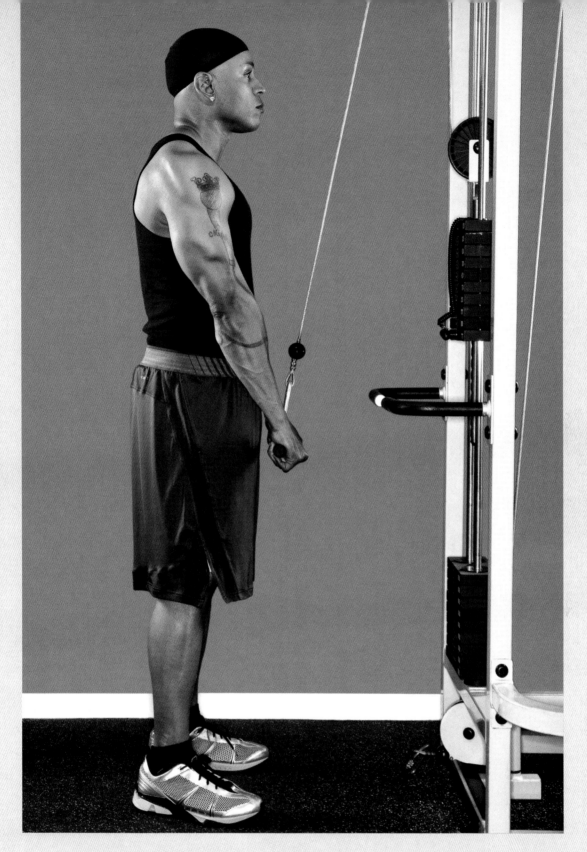

Cable Pressdown: Stand in front of a high cable pulley and grasp the straight-bar attachment with an overhand grip. With your knees a bit bent, lean forward slightly at the waist and position your elbows close to your sides, your lower arms parallel to the floor. Flex your triceps and press the bar down toward the floor until your arms are fully extended, hold for a brief count, and return to the start position, stopping just before the weight stack touches down.

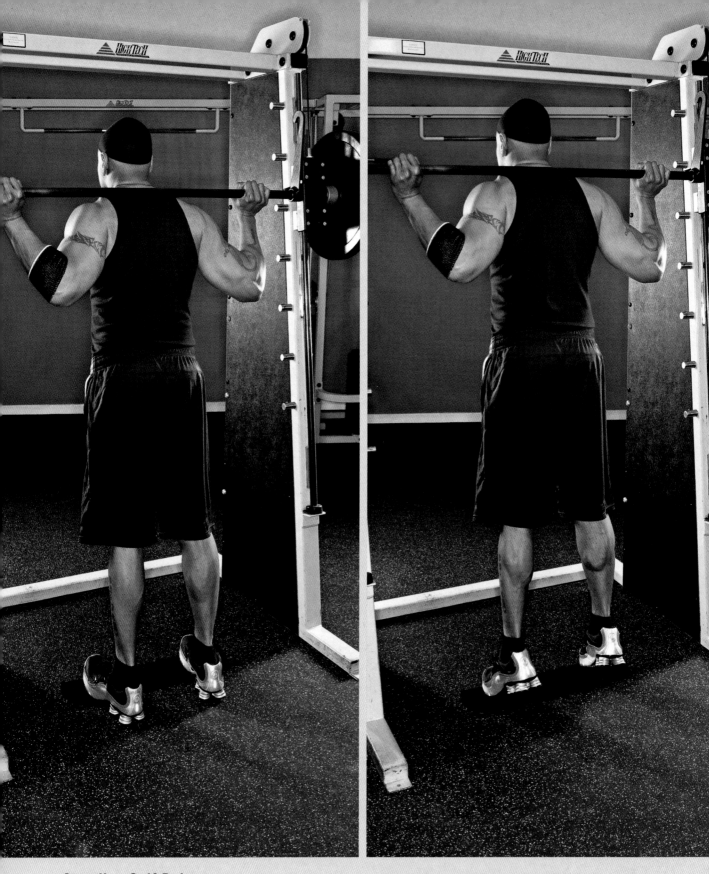

Standing Calf Raise: Step into a Smith machine or a standing calf machine, body erect, knees straight, the bar securely atop your shoulders, and the balls of your feet on the footrests. Press up with your calves to unrack the weight, then lower your heels to the floor. After a good stretch, press up onto your toes as high as possible, squeeze, and repeat.

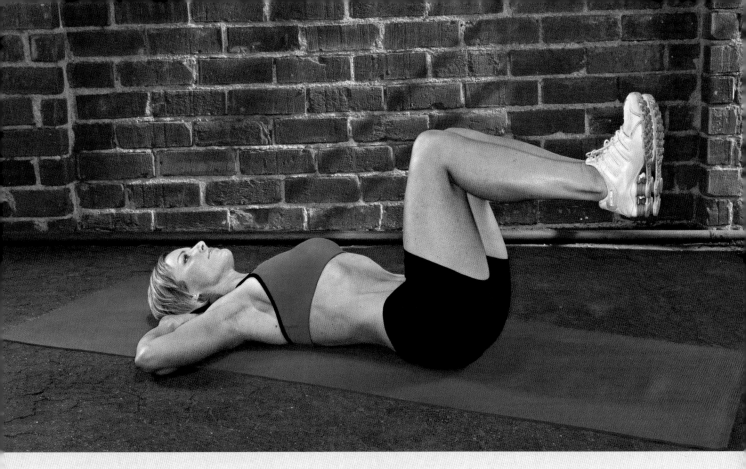

Crunch: Lie faceup on the floor with your legs at a 90-degree angle. Place your hands behind your head with your fingertips touching to support your head and your elbows out to your sides. Slowly curl your upper body, raising your shoulder blades off the floor as your bring your chest and shoulders toward the ceiling. At the top, squeeze your abs before returning to the start position.

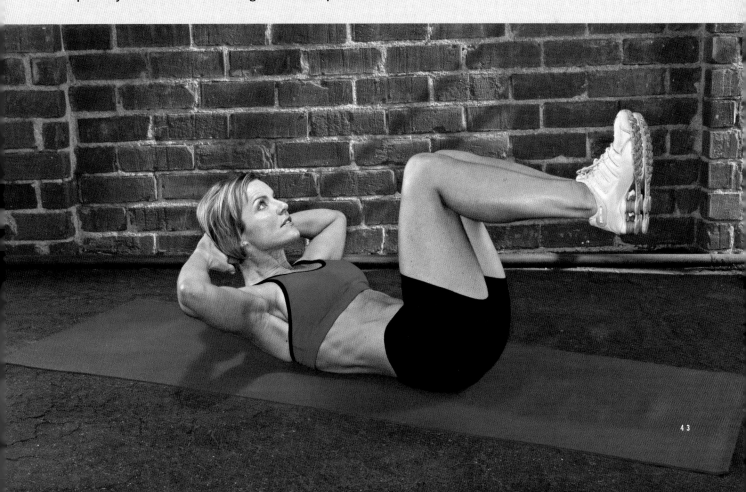

PHASE 2:
Weeks 3 and 4
Going High and Low

Phase 2 brings on the next level of training, where you split your upper and lower body out into two different workouts. This system allows you to better target each section with more volume (i.e., more exercises, sets, and/or reps) and not overly fatigue yourself.

PHASE 2 TRAINING SPLIT

DAY	MODE
1	Upper body, abs, steady-state cardio
2	Lower body, calves, abs, interval cardio
3	Rest
4	Upper body, abs, steady-state cardio
5	Lower body, calves, abs, interval cardio
6	Rest
7	Rest

The upper-body workout covers your chest, back, shoulders, traps, biceps, and triceps, while the lower-body session takes aim at your quadriceps (the large muscle on the front of your thighs), hamstrings (the muscles on the backs of your thighs), glutes (your butt), and your calves (the muscles on the backs of your lower legs). The abdominals and core, which keep you stable during complex movements and allow you to balance, are a part of both the upper- and lower-body days.

Your cardio sessions will grow more strenuous during this phase, as we start to kick your fat-burning engines into high gear. In addition to two slow and easy (steady-state or steady-pace) sessions, similar to the type you did in Weeks 1 and 2, you'll add interval cardio to your repertoire.

What is interval cardio? It's a technique in which you cycle bouts of high-intensity activity (such as sprints) with lower-intensity activity (such as a fast walk or light jog). Research shows that this type of fast-and-slow cycled training tends to burn more body fat than cardio done at a steady pace. However, we keep steady-state cardio in the mix because you can quickly burn yourself out with high-intensity cardio, so the variety is key to keeping your body running at peak efficiency.

For your two 20-minute interval workouts these 2 weeks, you'll go at a steady pace for 5 minutes, then start interspersing 1 minute at a fast pace with 1 minute at a slow (recovery) pace. Return to a steady, rhythmic pace for the final 5 minutes.

Phase 2 Workouts

You'll do each of the following workouts twice this week and next; for instance, the upper-body session can be done on Monday and Thursday, while the lower-body workout can be completed on Tuesday and Friday.

Days 1 and 4: Upper Body

Exercise	Sets	Reps
Smith Bench Press	3	8–12
Seated Cable Row	3	8–12
Standing Overhead Press	2	8–12
Barbell Curl	3	8–12
Cable Pressdown (page 41)	3	8–12
Cable Crunch	3	8–12

Days 2 and 5: Lower Body

Exercise	Sets	Reps
Smith Squat	3	8–12
Leg Press (page 33)	3	8–12
Dumbbell Stepup	2	8–12
Leg Extension (page 34)	3	8–12
Barbell Lunge	3	8–12
Lying Leg Curl (page 35)	3	8–12
Seated Calf Raise	2	8–12

In both workouts, rest 1 minute between sets; does not include warmup sets.

Cardio: You'll perform two 30-minute steady-state workouts (slow and easy) on Days 1 and 4 and two 20-minute interval cardio workouts on Days 2 and 5, for a total of four cardio sessions per week. Do your cardio after your weight sessions for best results.

EXERCISE INSTRUCTIONS

Note: All new exercises introduced in Phase 2 are on the following pages; the other descriptions can be found in Phase 1, as they carry over.

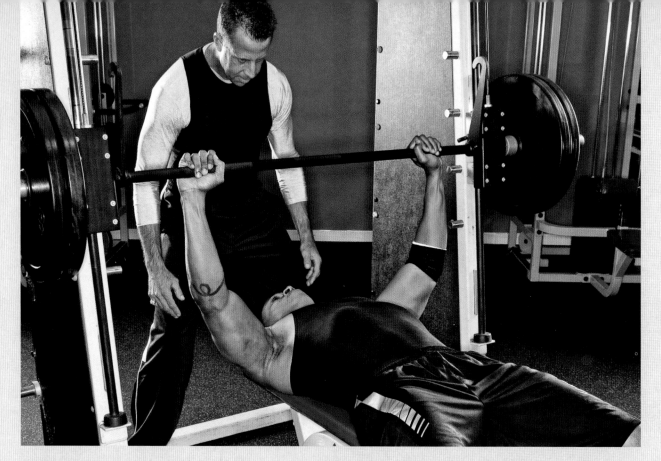

Smith Bench Press: Place a bench centered inside a Smith machine. Grasp the bar with a wide, overhand grip. Rotate the bar to unrack it. Slowly lower the bar to your chest, pausing when the bar is just about an inch away from your pecs, then powerfully press the bar back up to full arm extension and repeat.

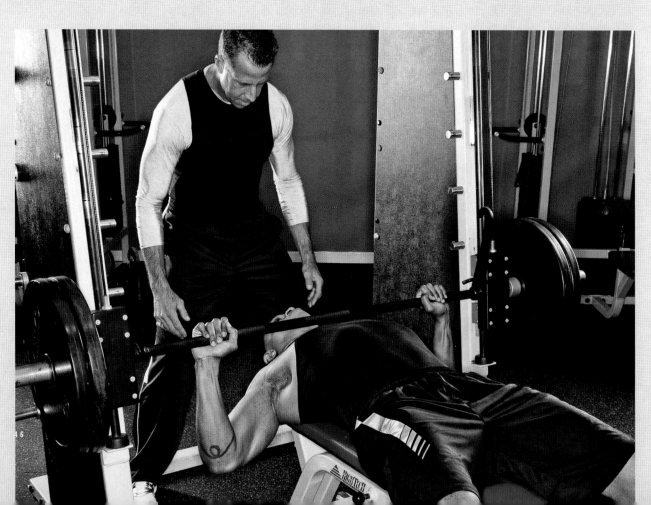

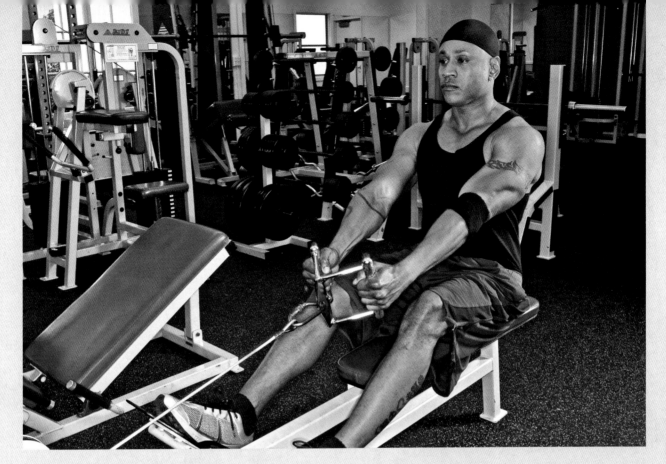

Seated Cable Row: Attach a close-grip handle to the seated cable row machine and sit upright on the bench facing the weight stack. Place your feet against the foot platform with your knees slightly bent. Reach forward to grasp the handle while keeping your back flat and chest up. Lean back until your torso is erect and your arms are fully extended. Pull the handle toward your midsection, your elbows in close to the sides of your body, and when the handle reaches your abdomen, hold for 1 to 2 seconds before slowly returning to the start position.

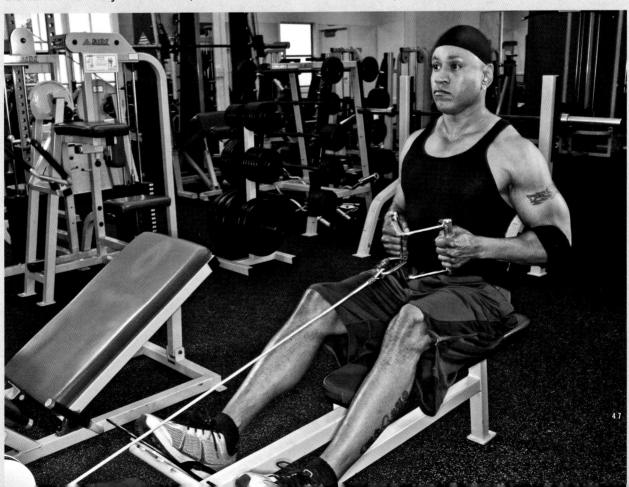

47

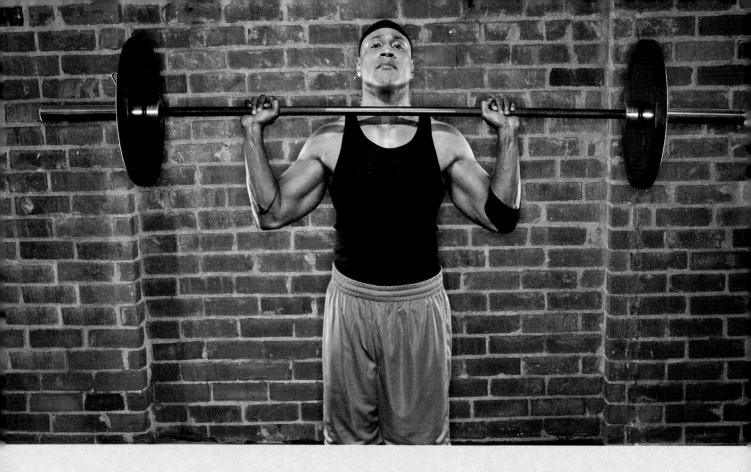

Standing Overhead Press: Carefully unrack the bar and hold it at shoulder level. In a smooth, strong motion, press the bar straight up to just short of elbow lockout, squeeze, and then lower the bar under control to the start position.

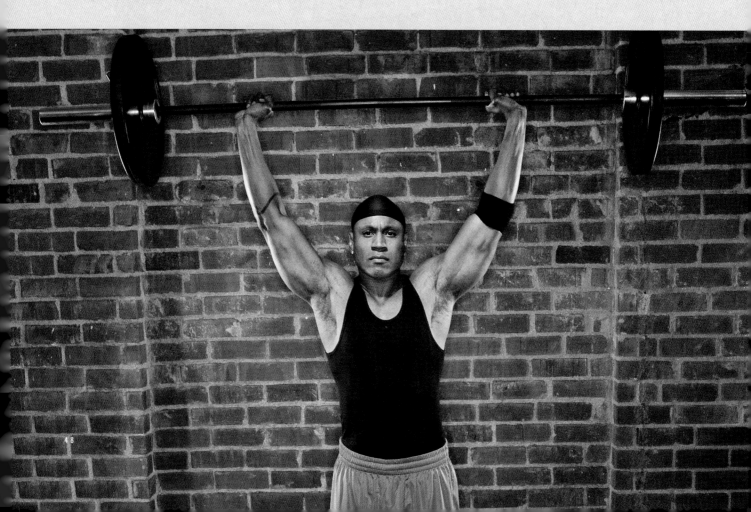

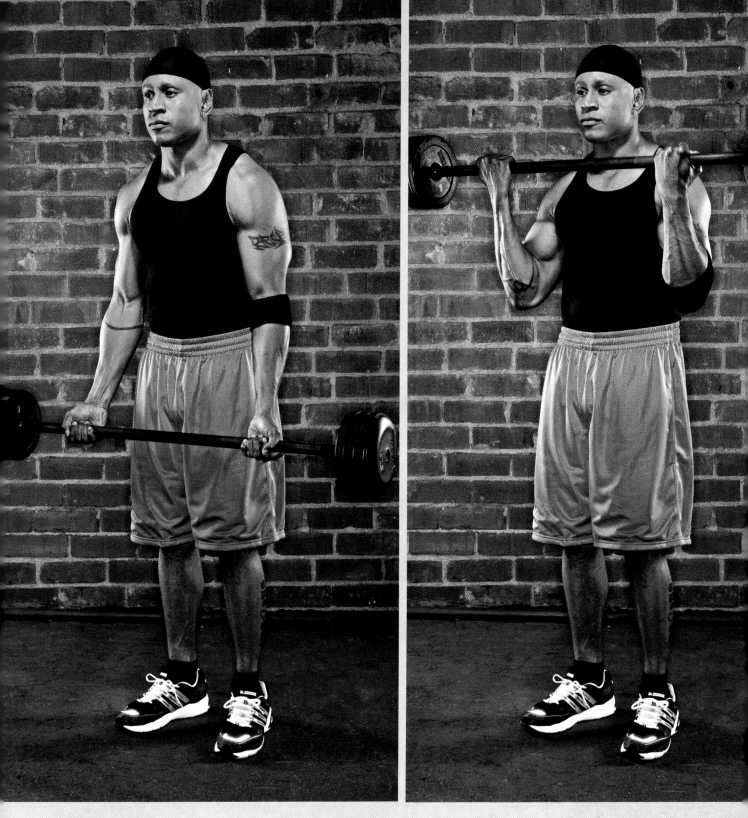

Barbell Curl: Stand holding a barbell with an underhand grip, arms extended. Contract your biceps to curl the bar toward your chest, keeping your elbows at your sides. Hold and squeeze at the top, then slowly return the bar along the same path.

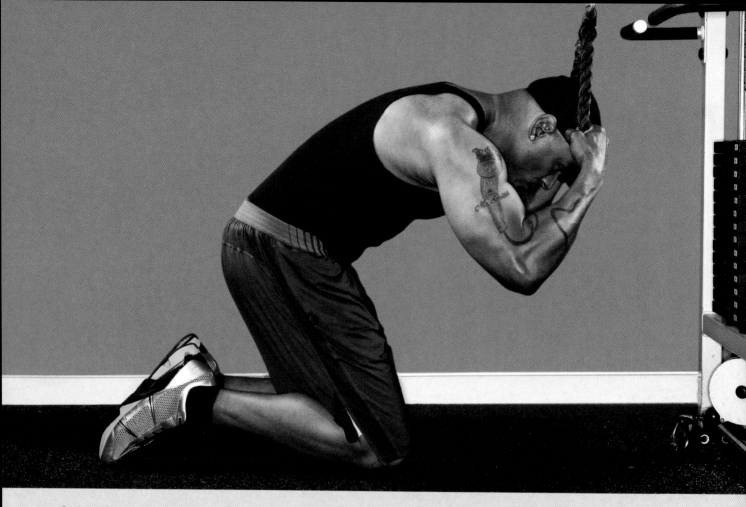

Cable Crunch: Kneel in front of a cable machine and grasp a rope attachment with both hands. With your lower arms aside your head, crunch down, taking your elbows toward the floor. Pause, then slowly return to the start position.

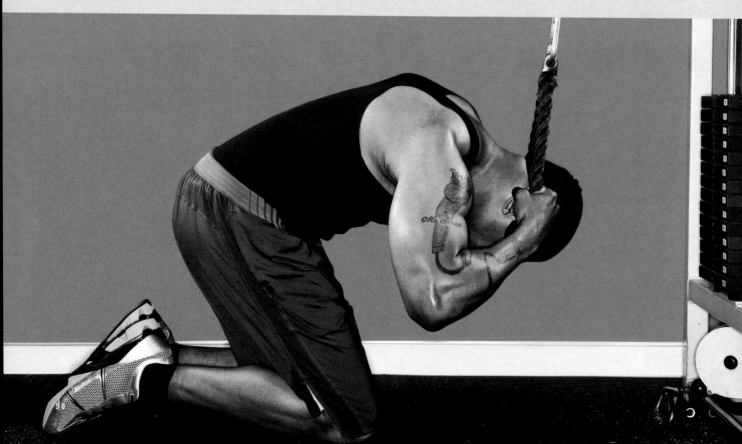

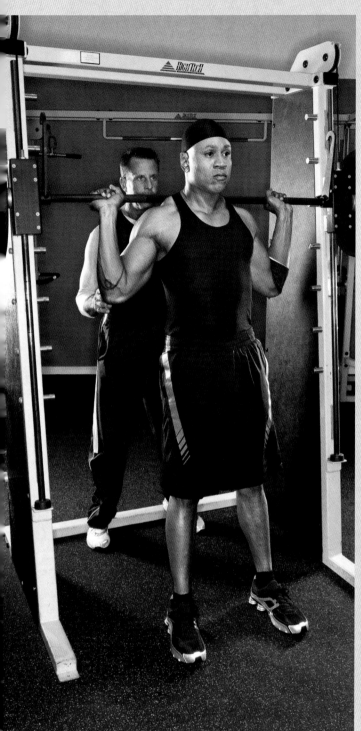
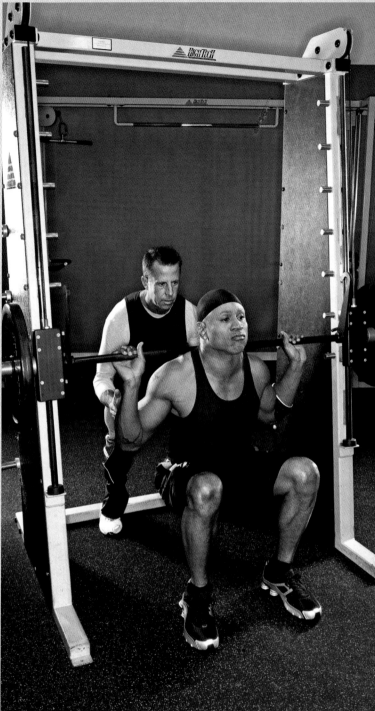

Smith Squat: Stand inside a Smith machine with the bar across your upper back and your feet planted just outside shoulder width, toes pointed out slightly. With your chest up, back flat, abs tight, and eyes focused forward, bend your knees and hips as if sitting in a chair until your thighs are parallel to the floor. Reverse the motion by driving through your heels and shifting your hips forward to return to the start position.

Scooter's Tip

If you want to lose weight and get in shape, you have to weight train. Doing cardio is only part of the equation. You have to get comfortable being uncomfortable, and then you'll see great results.

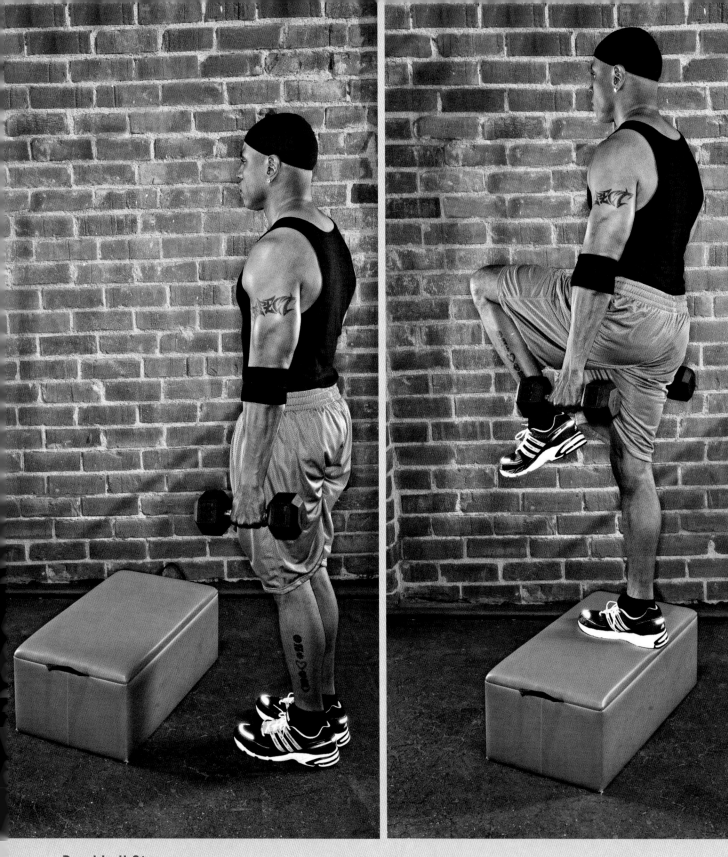

Dumbbell Stepup: Place a knee-high step in front of you (knee height is ideal) and grasp a dumbbell in each hand. Stand with your feet in a comfortable stance. Step forward with one leg onto the step and drive through that thigh to elevate your body. Bring the trailing leg to the top of the step and stand on the box, then step back with the opposite leg to the floor and lower yourself. Repeat the sequence with the opposite leg leading. That's 1 rep.

Scooter's Tip

"There is no impossible, only possible." Keep those words echoing in your head.
They're important, and they keep me and LL going when it gets hard.

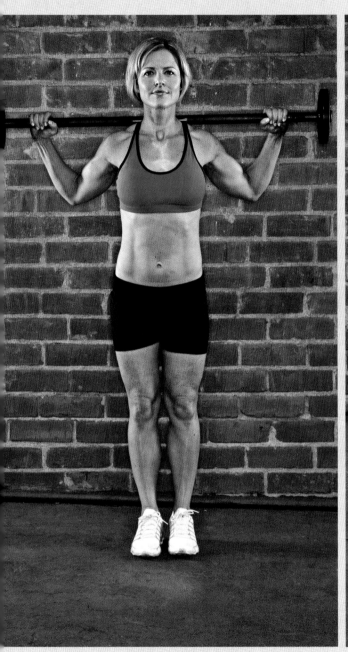
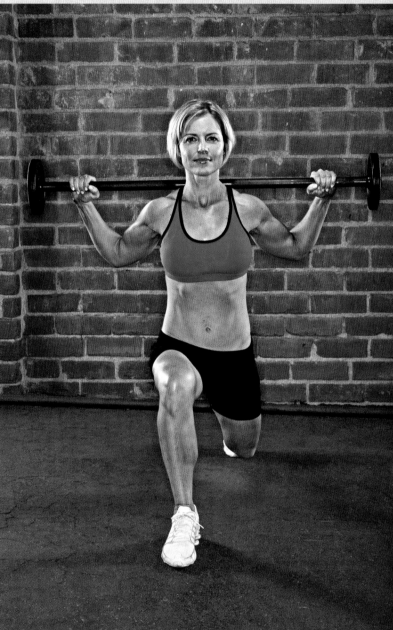

Barbell Lunge: Holding a barbell across your upper back, step forward with one foot. Bend both knees to lower yourself, making sure your front knee doesn't extend past your toes. Stop just short of your rear knee touching the floor and reverse directions, driving through the heel of your forward foot to return to the start position.

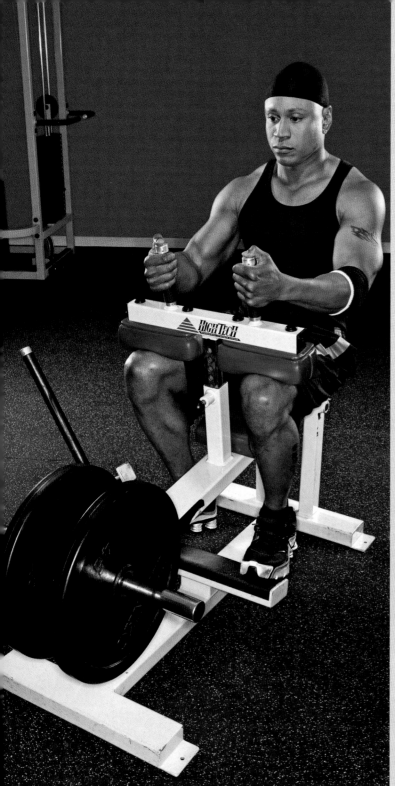
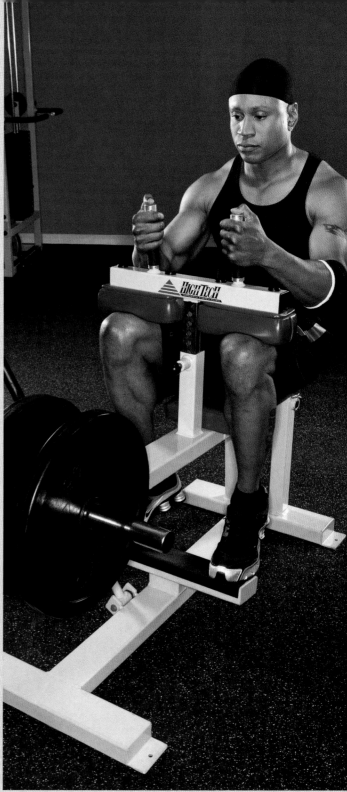

Seated Calf Raise: Sit in a seated calf machine with the balls of your feet on the footrests and the pads secured across your lower quads. Press up with your calves to unrack the weight, then lower your heels to the floor. After a good stretch, press up onto your toes as high as possible, squeeze, and repeat.

PHASE 3:
Weeks 5 and 6
Threes Are Wild

For Phase 3, you'll further hone your training split, dividing the body into three parts. This approach allows for more specialization—in other words, more specific attention to each individual muscle group.

Why is this specialization important? One reason is the opportunity to lift heavier weights for every muscle. Think about it: At the start of your workout, you're fresh and ready to take on the world. But by the end, you're likely flagging, which means whatever you save until last will not get the same level of benefit.

Another reason is the fact that your muscles are multitiered; it takes a number of different movements to target all of their areas directly. For example, your chest (or pectoral muscles, in technical parlance) should actually be thought of as three separate sections—the upper, middle, and lower pecs. Each of those areas can be more succinctly trained with incline, flat-bench, and decline presses and flies, respectively. Compound that by the number of body parts you need to incorporate, and a session trying to incorporate all the nuances of each would start to run into 2, 3 hours or more!

In addition to splitting your body into three, you'll also up the ante in your cardio, adding 5 minutes each to both your steady-state and interval sessions. We've paired intervals with your upper body, which we recommend sticking with, as the intensity required of those may prove to be too much if you try them after a hard leg workout. (Of course, if you choose to pair interval cardio and legs anyway, you'll probably flash back to our advice—right about the time you're trying to negotiate a set of stairs the next day and feel the sweet sting of muscle soreness on every step up. You've been warned.)

Phase 3 Workouts

You'll do each of the following workouts twice these 2 weeks, as laid out below.

PHASE 3 TRAINING SPLIT

DAY	MODE
1	Chest, shoulders, triceps, interval cardio
2	Legs, steady-state cardio
3	Back, biceps, abs, calves
4	Rest
5	Chest, shoulders, triceps, interval cardio
6	Legs, steady-state cardio
7	Back, biceps, abs, calves

EXERCISE INSTRUCTIONS

Note: All new exercises introduced in Phase 3 are on the following pages; the other descriptions can be found in Phases 1 and 2, as they carry over.

Days 1 and 5: Chest, Shoulders, Triceps

Exercise	Sets	Reps
Dumbbell Bench Press	3	8–12
Incline Cable Fly	3	8–12
Weighted Dip	2	8–12
Upright Row	3	8–12
Seated Overhead Dumbbell Press	3	8–12
Cable Lateral Raise	2	8–12
Cable Kickback	3	8–12
Reverse-Grip Pressdown	3	8–12
Bench Dip	2	8–12
Overhead Cable Extension	2	8–12

Days 2 and 6: Legs

Exercise	Sets	Reps
Barbell Squat	3	8–12
Leg Press (page 33)	3	8–12
Hack Squat	2	8–12
Leg Extension (page 34)	3	8–12
Barbell Lunge (page 53)	3	8–12
Lying Leg Curl (page 35)	3	8–12
Standing Calf Raise (page 42)	2	8–12
Seated Calf Raise (page 54)	2	8–12

Days 3 and 7: Back, Biceps, Abs, Calves

Exercise	Sets	Reps
Straight-Arm Pulldown	3	8–12
Dumbbell Pullover	3	8–12
Seated Cable Row (page 47)	3	8–12
Dumbbell Curl	3	8–12
Incline Dumbbell Curl	2	8–12
Dumbbell Preacher Curl	2	8–12
Hanging Leg Raise	3	to failure
Weighted Crunch	3	8–12
Standing Calf Raise (page 42)	3	8–12

Rest 1½ minutes between all sets in both workouts; does not include warmup sets.

Cardio: You'll perform two 35-minute interval cardio workouts with the chest, shoulders, and triceps sessions and two 25-minute steady-state cardio workouts with the leg sessions, for a total of four cardio workouts per week. Do your cardio after your weight sessions for best results.

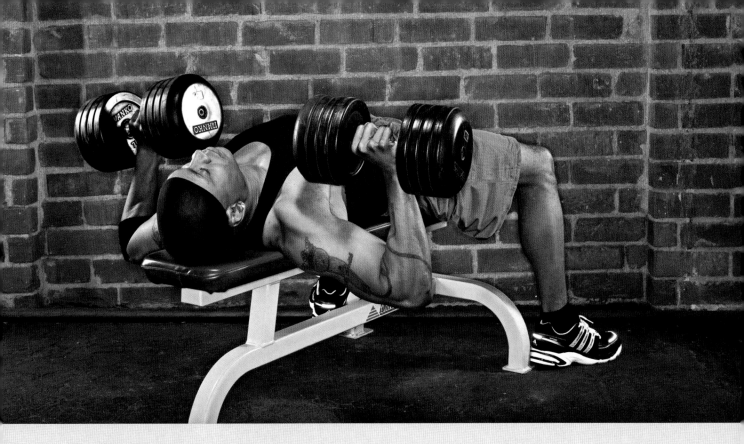

Dumbbell Bench Press: Lie faceup on the bench with your feet flat on the floor. Hold a dumbbell in each hand just outside your shoulders. Powerfully press the dumbbells upward toward the ceiling, stopping when the dumbbells are an inch or so away from each other, then slowly return to the start position and repeat.

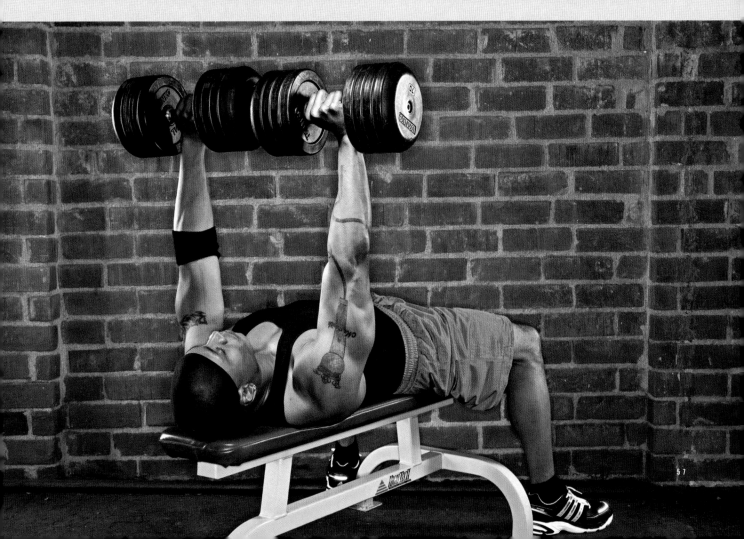

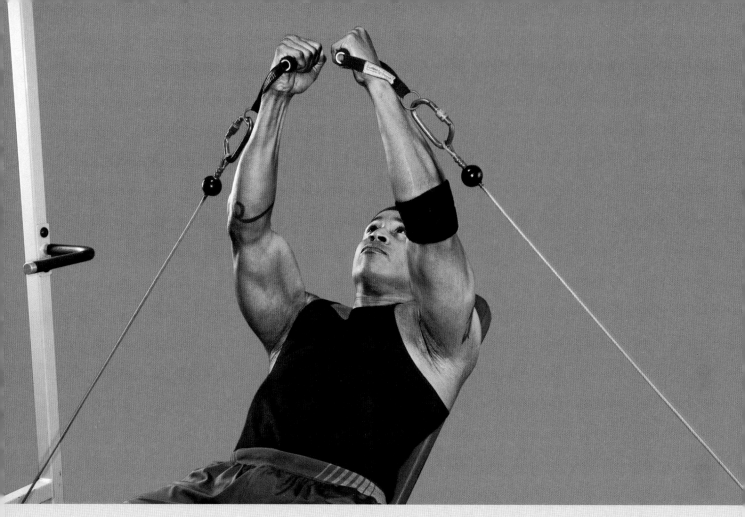

Incline Cable Fly: Adjust a bench inside a cable crossover so that the incline of the bench is roughly 30 to 45 degrees. Lie faceup with your feet flat on the floor. Hold a D-handle in each hand with a neutral grip and extend your arms above your chest. Bend your elbows slightly. Slowly lower the handles in a wide arc out to your sides, keeping your elbows locked in the slightly bent position throughout the range of motion. Stop when your elbows reach shoulder level before reversing the motion.

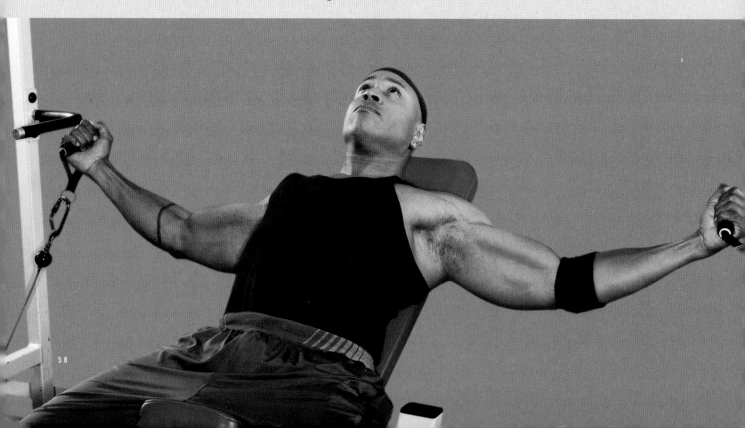

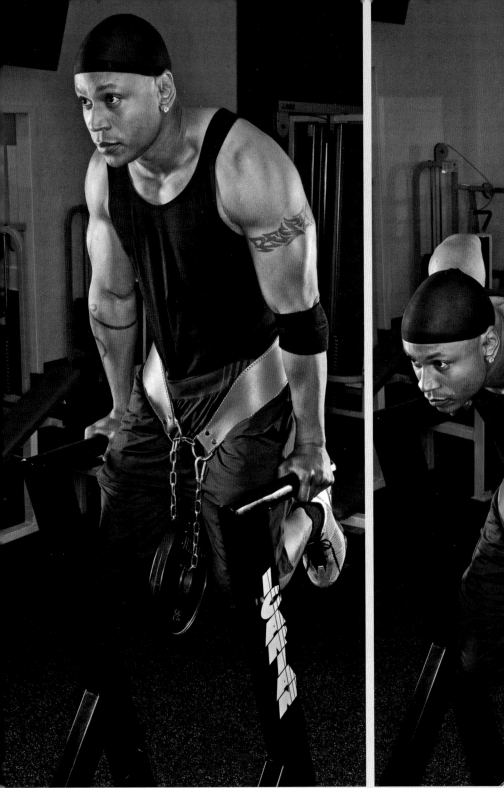
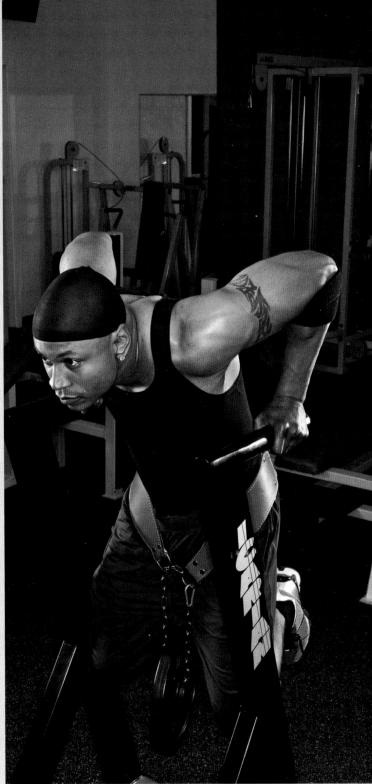

Weighted Dip: With weight hanging around your waist, grasp the dip bars with your arms extended. Lean forward and bend your knees while keeping your legs crossed. Keep your elbows out to your sides as you bend them to lower your body until your upper arms are about parallel to the floor. Press your hands into the bars to extend your arms and raise your body back up.

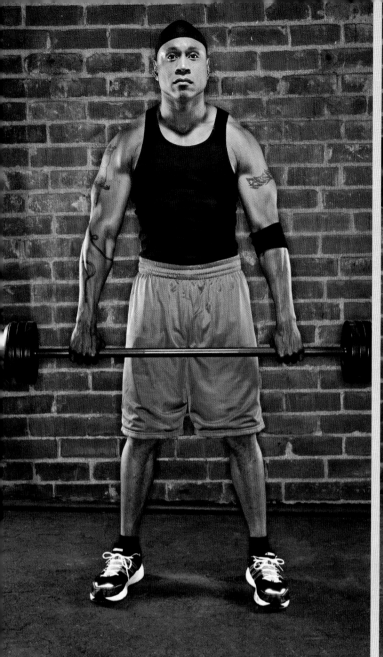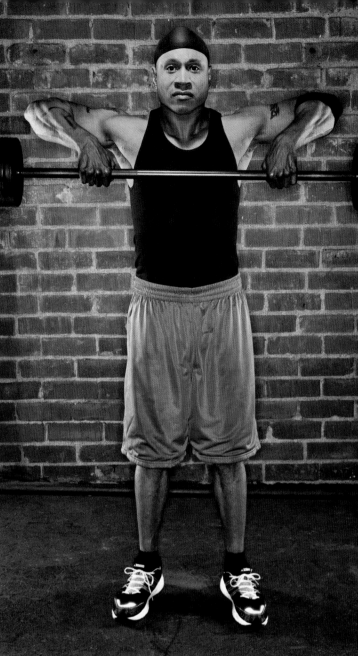

Upright Row: With your feet shoulder-width apart, stand erect holding a barbell in front of your thighs with a wide, overhand grip. Flex your shoulders and pull the barbell straight up toward your chin, keeping the bar close to your body during the entire movement. Maintain an erect torso and the natural curve in your spine throughout the exercise. In the top position, your elbows will be high and pointing out to your sides. Hold there for a second before slowly lowering to the start position.

Scooter's Tip

Don't complain—train. If you cheat yourself, you're going to cheat your results.

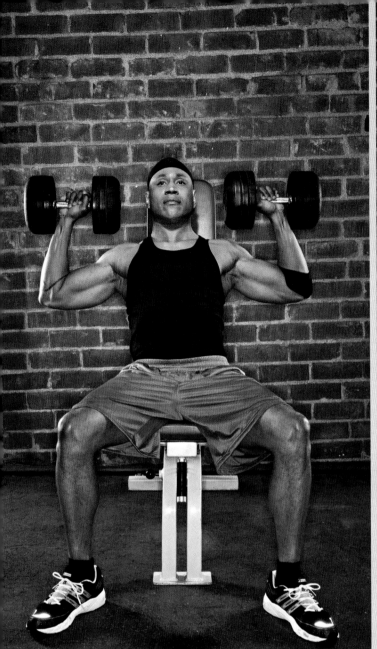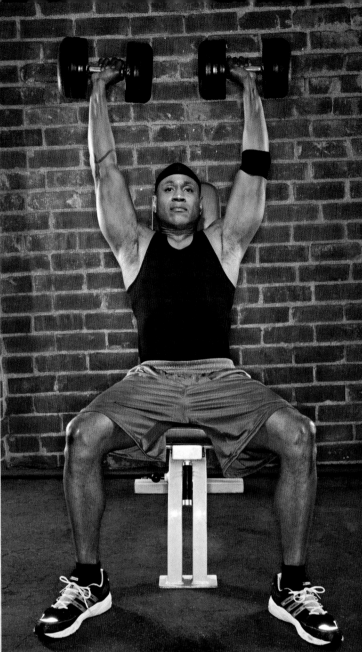

Seated Overhead Dumbbell Press: Sit on a low-back bench, holding a dumbbell in each hand above shoulder level with a pronated grip (palms facing forward). Keeping your shoulders back, press the dumbbells overhead in an arc, but don't let the weights touch at the top. Slowly lower to the start position and repeat.

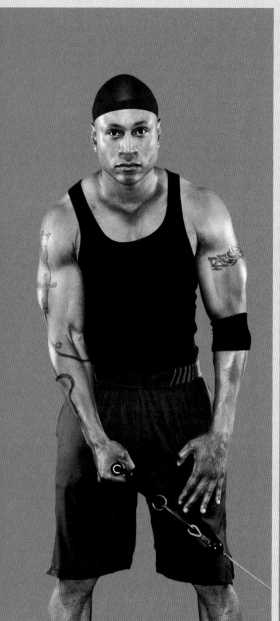
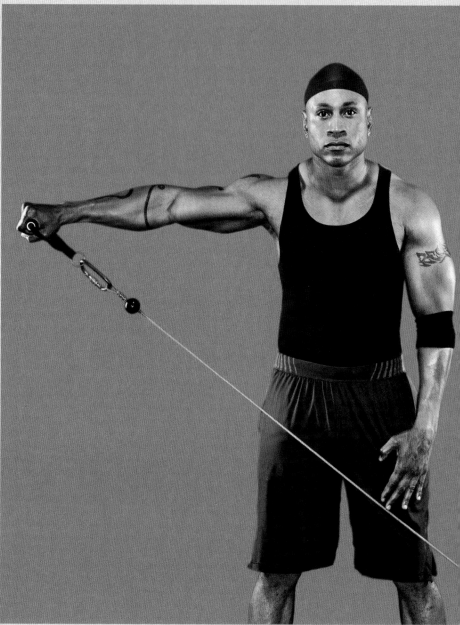

Cable Lateral Raise: Stand sideways to a low cable pulley with your feet shoulder-width apart. Grasp a D-handle with your hand opposite the machine. Without using momentum, raise the handle out to your side in a wide arc, keeping your elbow and hand moving together in the same plane. Raise your arm just above shoulder level and hold momentarily in the peak contracted position, then slowly lower it along the same path and repeat for reps.

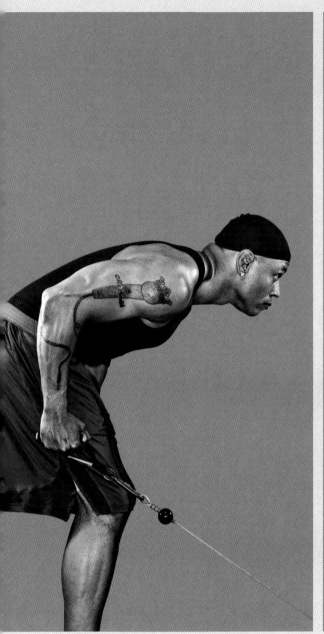 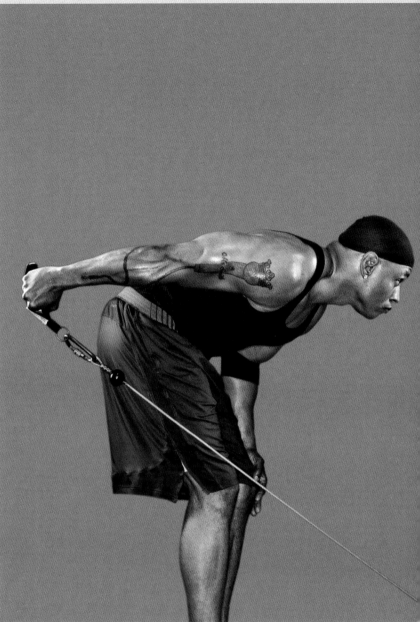

Cable Kickback: Grasp the handle on the lower pulley cable and align the working-side shoulder with the pulley. Bend over until your upper body is almost parallel to the floor and raise your upper arm to a point parallel to your torso, pressing it into your side. Holding your upper arm in place, kick your lower arm straight back to full extension. Don't allow your elbow to drop as you return to the start position.

Reverse-Grip Pressdown: Stand in front of a high cable pulley and grasp the straight-bar attachment with an underhand grip. With your knees a bit bent, lean forward slightly at the waist and position your elbows close to your sides, your lower arms parallel to the floor. Flex your triceps and press the bar down toward the floor until your arms are fully extended, hold for a brief count, and return to the start position, stopping just before the weight stack touches down.

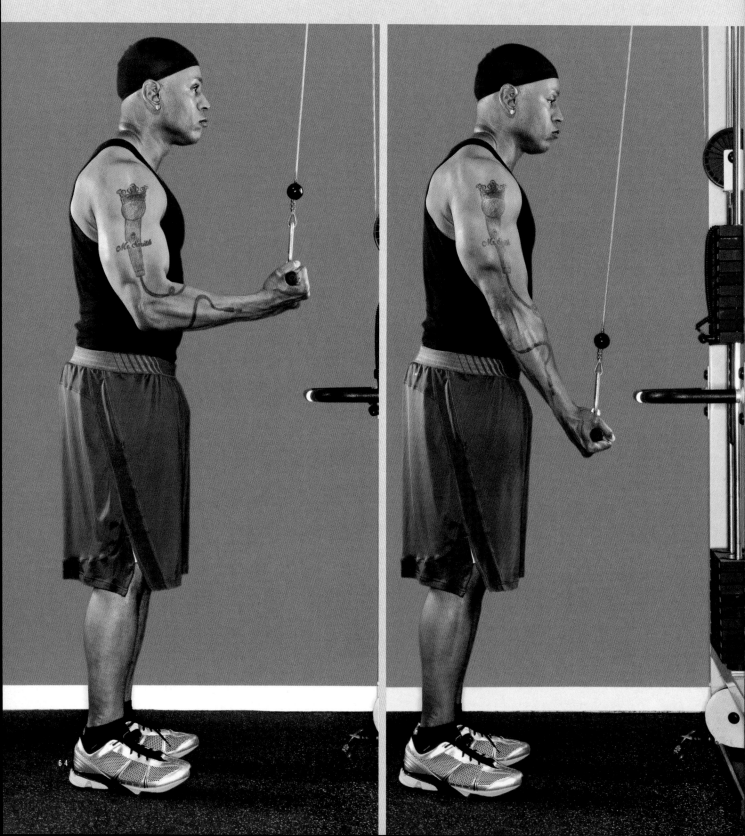

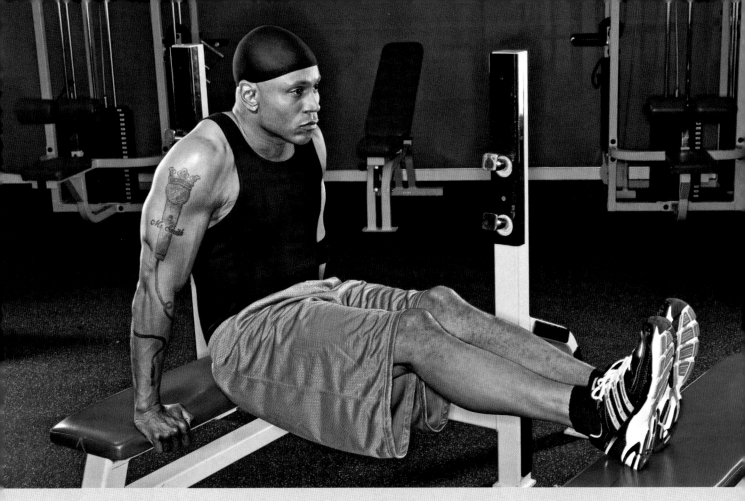

Bench Dip: Place two benches a few feet apart and parallel to each other and sit on the middle edge of one bench facing the other. Place your hands just outside your hips on the bench, cupping the bench with your fingers, and set your heels on the opposite bench, pressing yourself upward so that your body forms an "L" in the top position. Slowly lower your glutes toward the floor until your arms form 90-degree angles. Pause, then forcefully press yourself back up to the start position. To increase difficulty, have a partner place a weight in your lap.

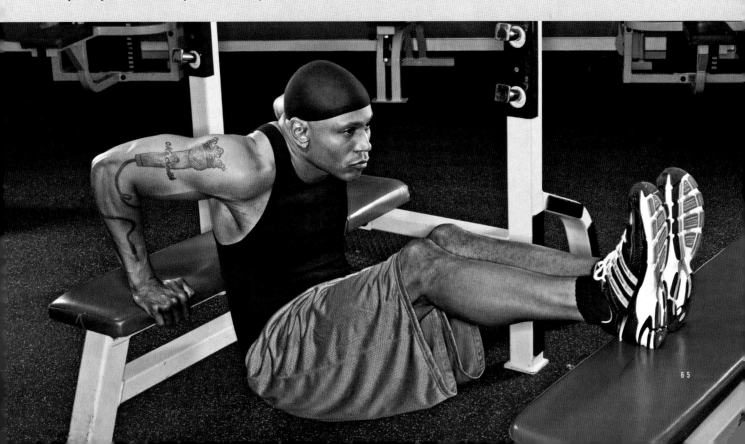

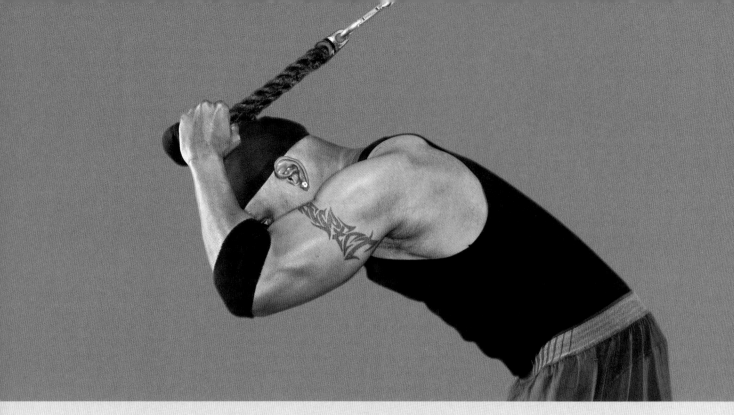

Overhead Cable Extension: Attach a rope to a high-cable pulley, then grasp it with a neutral, shoulder-width grip and face away from the stack. Take a step out with one foot and lean forward at the waist 30 to 45 degrees, keeping your abs tight, eyes forward, back straight, and upper arms almost parallel to the floor. Moving only your lower arms, extend them out in front of you until they are parallel to the floor. Squeeze your triceps hard before returning to the start position.

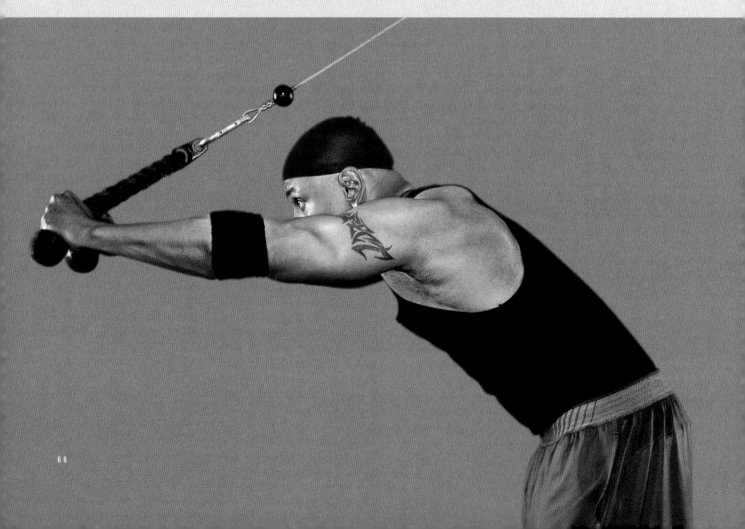

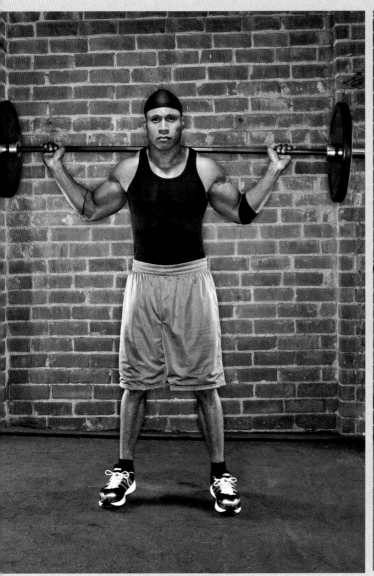
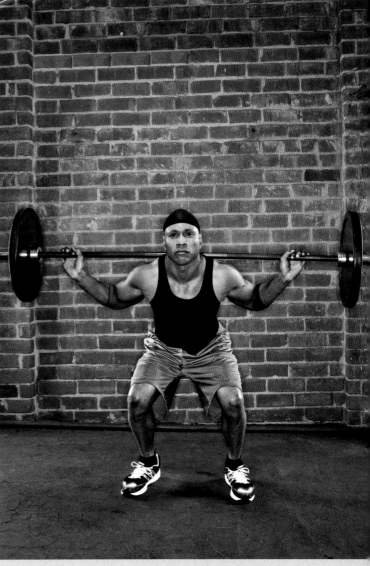

Barbell Squat: Stand holding a bar across your upper back with your feet about shoulder-width apart, knees slightly bent, and your toes turned out slightly. Keeping your head neutral, abs tight, and torso erect, bend at the knees and hips to slowly lower your body as if you were going to sit down in a chair. Pause when your knees reach a 90-degree angle, then forcefully drive through your heels, extending at your hips and knees until you arrive at the standing position.

Hack Squat (not pictured): Step inside a hack squat machine, placing your shoulders and back against the pads. Place your feet narrow and low on the platform. Unhook the safety bars and slowly lower yourself into the bottom position, stopping when your legs are well beyond parallel to the platform. Pause, then forcefully press yourself upward to the start position, keeping your knees bent slightly at the top. Squeeze your thighs and glutes and begin the next repetition.

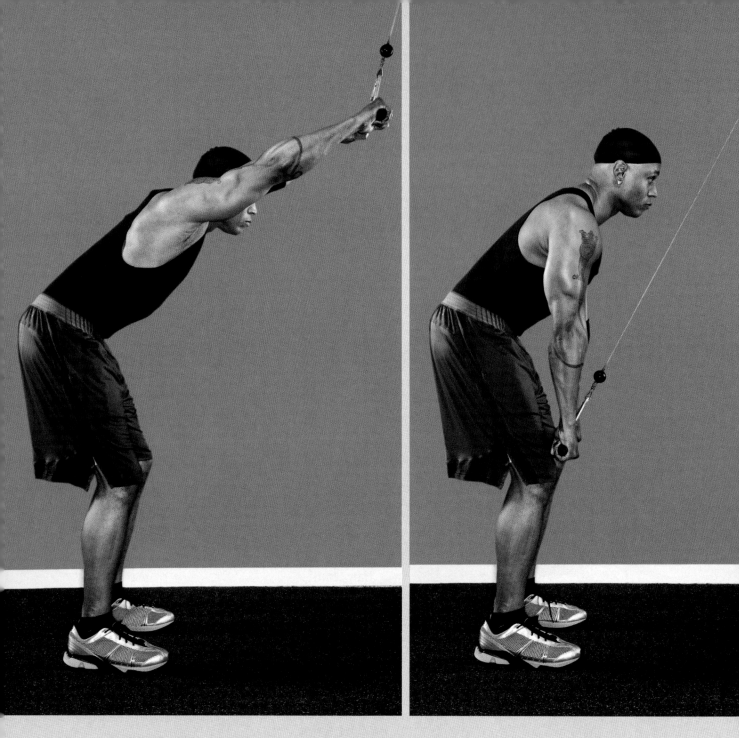

Straight-Arm Pulldown: Stand facing the weight stack at a lat-pulldown station with your feet shoulder-width apart. Reach up and grasp a standard lat-pulldown bar or long straight bar with an overhand (pronated) grip, hands shoulder-width apart, arms straight. Start with your arms extended and almost parallel to the floor. Keeping your arms straight, pull the bar down toward your thighs in a wide, sweeping arc, focusing on using just your lats as you pull. Squeeze your lats hard once the bar reaches your thighs and return to the start position in a smooth, controlled motion, stopping once your arms are parallel to the floor.

T-Bar Row (not pictured): With your arms fully extended, grasp the handles of a T-bar rowing machine with an overhand, palms-down grip. With your chest up and back flat, head in a neutral position, pull the handles toward you, keeping your elbows close to your body. Do not allow your upper body to rise in an effort to pull the weight upward. Hold the peak contracted position momentarily before slowly lowering the weight to the start position.

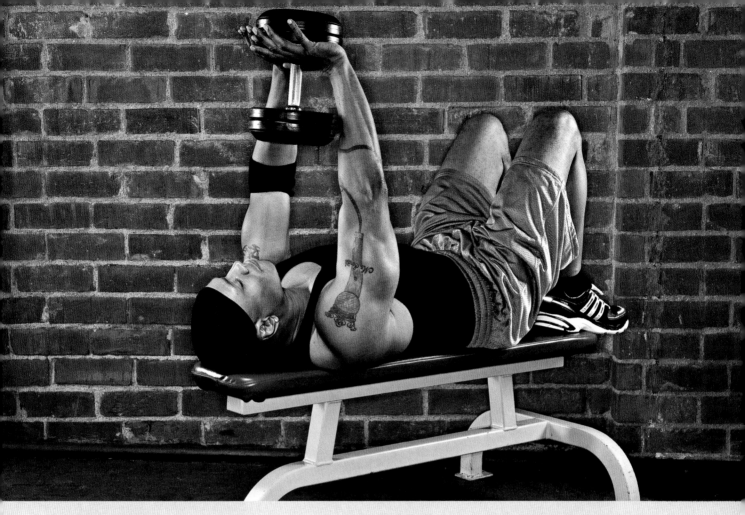

Dumbbell Pullover: Lie on a flat bench with your upper back, head, and neck supported by the bench, knees bent and feet on the bench. Hold a dumbbell with your arms extended above your face. Keeping your arms straight, slowly lower the dumbbell back toward the top of your head, feeling a good stretch in your chest. Pause, then forcefully reverse direction with the dumbbell, squeezing your pectorals at the top.

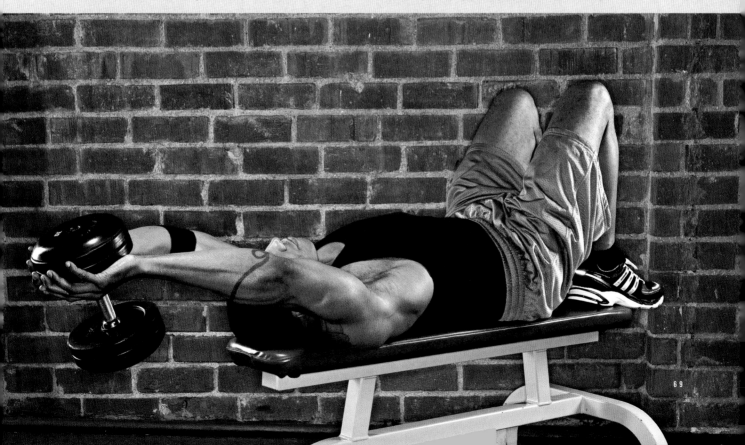

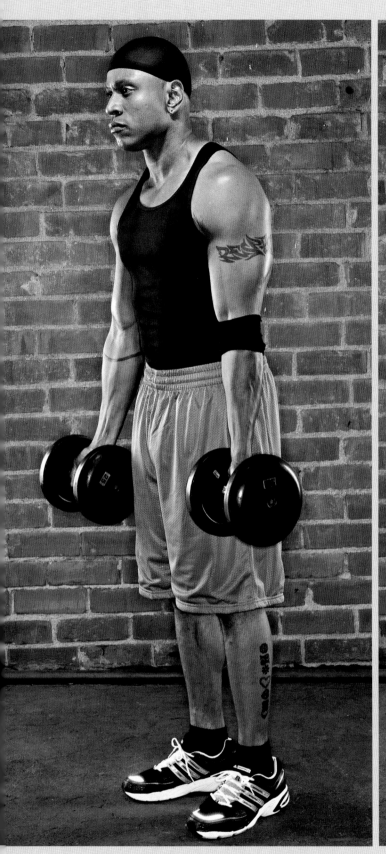
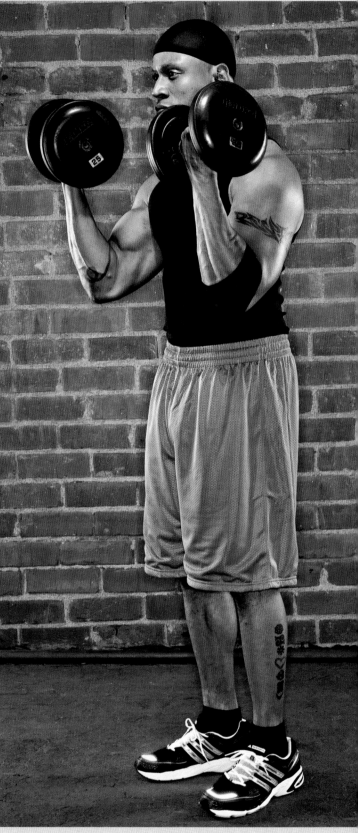

Dumbbell Curl: Stand holding a pair of dumbbells at your sides, arms extended. Contract your biceps to curl the dumbbells toward your shoulders, keeping your elbows at your sides. Hold and squeeze at the top, then slowly return the dumbbells along the same path.

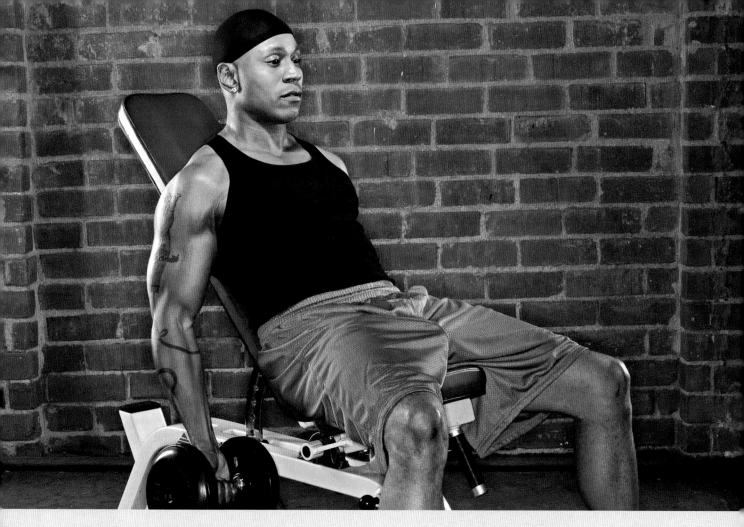

Incline Dumbbell Curl: Adjust an incline bench to about 45 to 60 degrees and sit back squarely against the bench, feet flat on the floor. Your arms should hang straight down by your sides, palms up. Keeping your shoulders back and upper arms in a fixed position perpendicular to the floor, curl the weights up so the dumbbells approach your shoulders. Squeeze your biceps hard at the top before slowly returning to the start position.

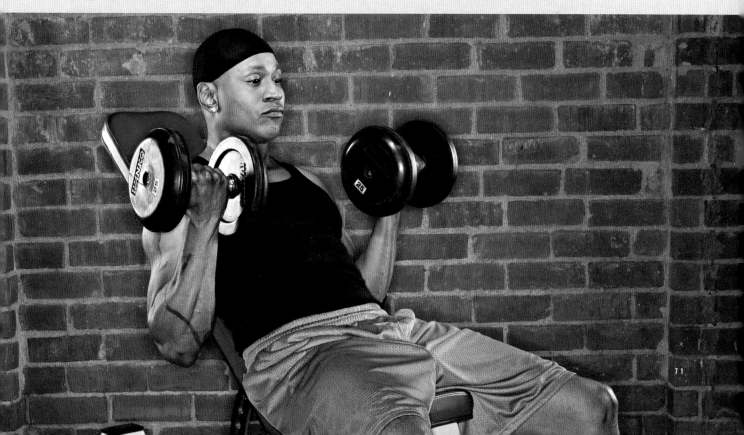

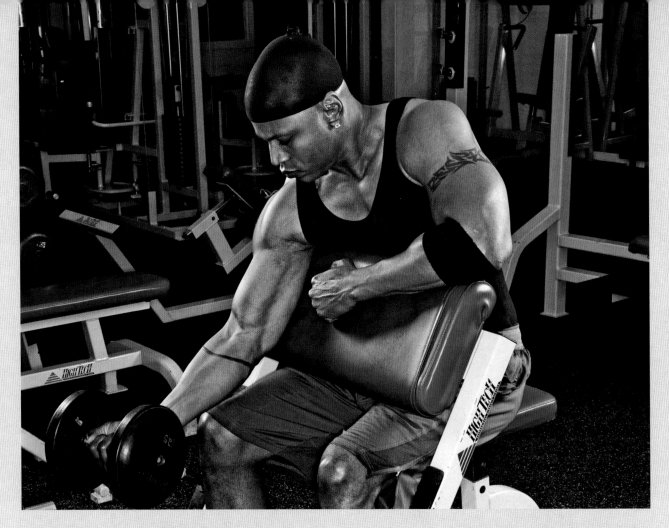

Dumbbell Preacher Curl: Grasp a dumbbell with an underhand grip and drape your arm over either a standing or seated preacher bench. Keeping your shoulder down and wrist flat and rigid, raise the dumbbell in an arc toward your face—stop just short of bringing your forearm perpendicular to the floor. Squeeze at the top, then return to the start position.

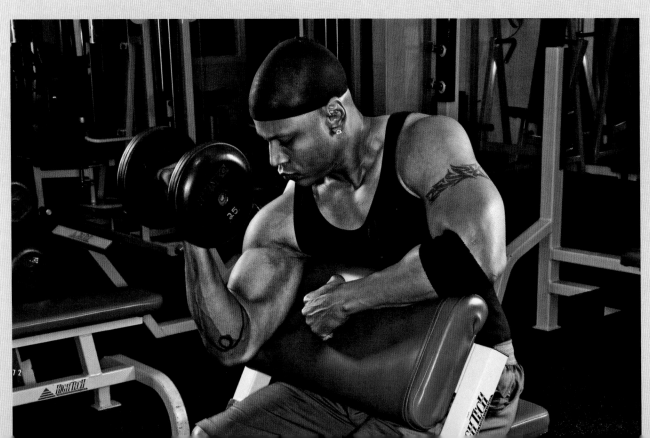

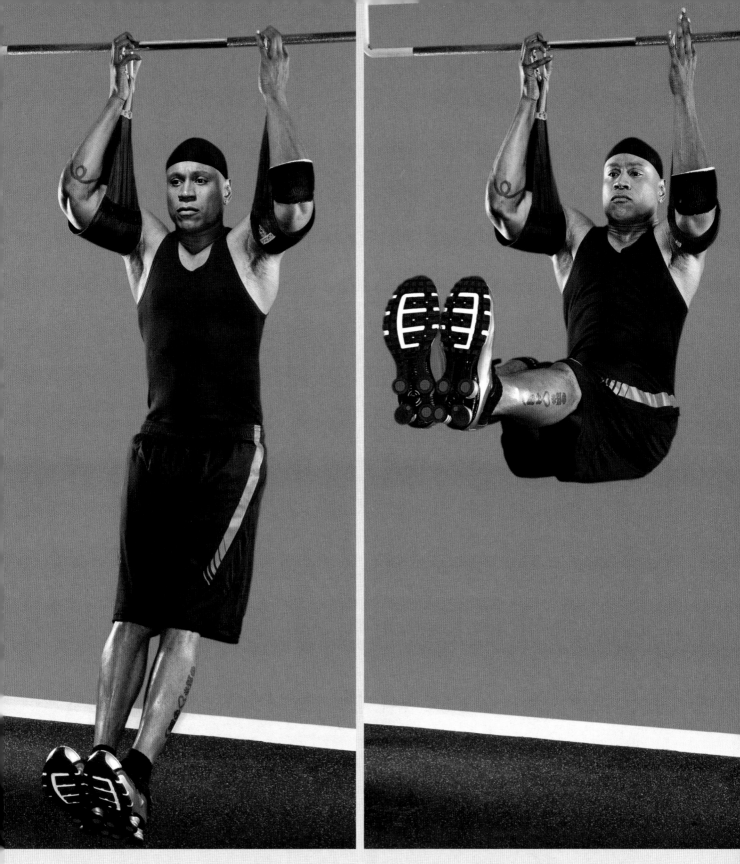

Hanging Leg Raise: Grasp an overhead bar and hang freely. Raise your legs straight up in front of you to hip level without using momentum. Pause for a 2-count, then return to the start position and repeat.

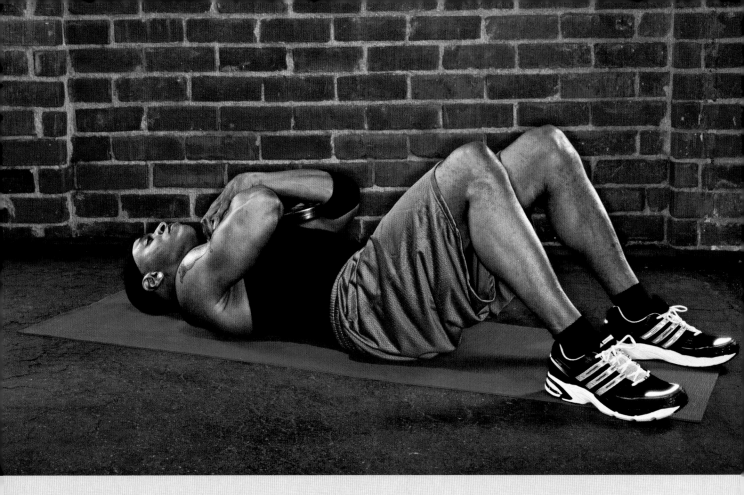

Weighted Crunch: Lie faceup on the floor with your legs bent and your feet flat on the floor. Hold a 10- or 25-pound weight plate on your chest with your elbows out to your sides. Slowly curl your upper body, raising your shoulder blades off the floor as you bring your chest and shoulders toward the ceiling. At the top, squeeze your abs before returning to the start position.

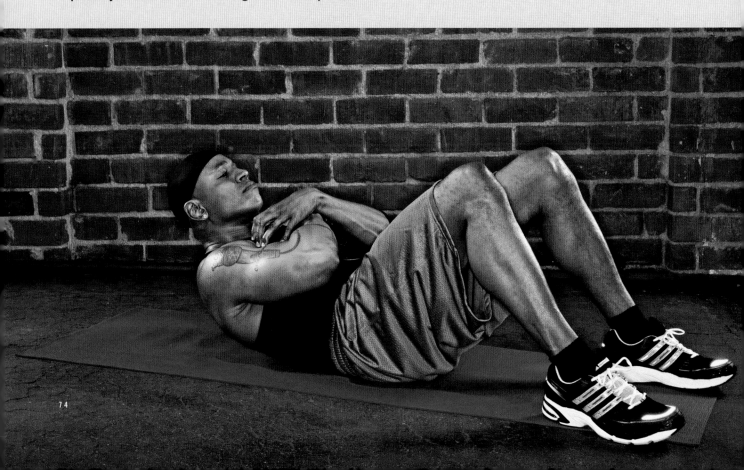

PHASE 4:
Weeks 7 and 8
The Drop Zone

Phase 4 brings on a challenging but effective new technique in drop sets. The idea is to push your muscles to their breaking point and then go beyond to ignite growth. The concept is relatively simple: You do reps as specified—for instance, 12—and when you get to that point, immediately drop the weight about 20 to 30 percent and continue doing reps until you can't possibly complete one more with proper form. The searing burn you'll feel will be almost unbearable, but stick with it—that's the sweet sting of progress. Hey, if training and having a great body were easy, every dude on the street would be ripped.

Take note this phase: While the weight workouts shift pretty dramatically, your cardio sessions will remain the same as they were in Phase 3. Trust me, the weight-training alterations will be more than enough for you to adjust to—you'll be happy to have at least your cardio stay status quo because even more dramatic changes are coming.

PHASE 4 TRAINING SPLIT

DAY	MODE
1	Chest, shoulders, triceps, abs, interval cardio
2	Legs, calves, back, biceps, forearms, abs, steady-state cardio
3	Rest
4	Chest, shoulders, traps, triceps, abs, interval cardio
5	Rest
6	Legs, back, biceps, abs, steady-state cardio
7	Rest

Phase 4 Workouts

You'll do each of the workouts once per week, making sure to never work out more than 2 days in a row without inserting a day of rest. For instance, you could train Monday, Tuesday, Thursday, and Saturday.

Day 1: Chest, Shoulders, Triceps, Abs

Exercise	Sets	Reps
Incline Bench Press*	4	12, 12, 8, 8
Flat-Bench Dumbbell Fly	3	12, 10, 8
Bench Dip (page 65)	3	12, 10, 8
Overhead Dumbbell Press* (page 61)	4	12, 12, 6, 6
Upright Row (page 60)	3	8, 6, 6
Cable Lateral Raise (page 62)	3	12, 12, 12
Close-Grip Bench Press	3	12, 12, 12
Rope Pressdown*	3	15, 10, 8
Cable Crunch (page 50)	3	To failure
superset with		
Hanging Leg Raise (page 73)	3	To failure

*Perform as a drop set; the reps listed are the number you do on that first set before you lighten the weight. On that first drop, continue until muscle failure. Rest 2 minutes between drop sets and 1 minute between all other sets.

Day 2: Legs, Calves, Back, Biceps, Forearms, Abs

Exercise	Sets	Reps
Leg Press* (page 33)	4	12, 12, 8, 6
Leg Extension (page 34)	3	10, 10, 8
Lying Leg Curl (page 35)	3	10, 10, 8
Romanian Deadlift	3	10, 10, 8
Seated Calf Raise (page 54)	4	25, 25, 12, 12
Lat Pulldown* (page 36)	3	12, 8, 8
Seated Cable Row (wide grip) (page 47)	3	12, 12, 12
Dumbbell Row	3	12, 12, 12
Barbell Curl* (page 49)	4	12, 10, 8, 6
Incline Dumbbell Curl (page 71)	3	10, 10, 8
One-Arm Cable Curl	3	10, 10, 8
Dumbbell Wrist Curl*	3	12, 10, 10
Hanging Knee Raise	3	To failure
Crunch (page 43)	2	15, 15

Day 3: Rest

Day 4: Chest, Shoulders, Traps, Triceps, Abs

Decline Bench Press*	3	12, 10, 8
Dumbbell Bench Press (page 57)	3	10, 8, 6
Pec-Deck Fly	3	10, 8, 6
Overhead Machine Press* (page 39)	4	12, 10, 8, 6
Dumbbell Lateral Raise	3	10, 8, 6
Dumbbell Front Raise	3	10, 10, 10
Barbell Shrug	3	6, 6, 6
Straight-Bar Cable Pressdown* (page 41)	3	10, 10, 8
Overhead Cable Extension (page 66)	3	10, 8, 6
Weighted Dip (page 59)	3	10, 8, 6
Hanging Knee Raise	3	To failure
Weighted Crunch (page 74)	2	To failure

Day 5: Rest

Day 6: Legs, Back, Biceps, Abs

Exercise	Sets	Reps
Smith Squat (page 51)	4	10, 10, 6, 6
Walking Lunge	3	10, 10, 8
Lying Leg Curl (page 35)	3	10, 10, 8
Romanian Deadlift	3	10, 10, 8
Standing Calf Raise* (page 42)	3	10, 12, 15
Bent-Over Barbell Row	3	10, 8, 6
Seated Cable Row (page 47)	3	10, 8, 6
Lat Pulldown (underhand grip) (page 36)	3	12, 12, 12
Dumbbell Curl* (page 70)	4	10, 8, 6, 6
Dumbbell Preacher Curl (page 72)	3	10, 8, 6
Crunch (page 43)	3	To failure
Hanging Leg Raise (page 73)	3	To failure

*Perform as a drop set; the reps listed are the number you do on that first set before you lighten the weight. On that first drop, continue until muscle failure. Rest 2 minutes between drop sets and 1 minute between all other sets.

Cardio: You'll perform two 35-minute interval cardio workouts with the Day 1 and Day 4 sessions, and two 25-minute steady-state cardio workouts with the Day 2 and Day 6 sessions, for a total of four cardio workouts per week. Do your cardio after your weight sessions for best results.

Day 7: Rest

EXERCISE INSTRUCTIONS

Note: All new exercises introduced in Phase 4 are on the following pages; the other descriptions can be found in Phases 1, 2, and 3, as they carry over.

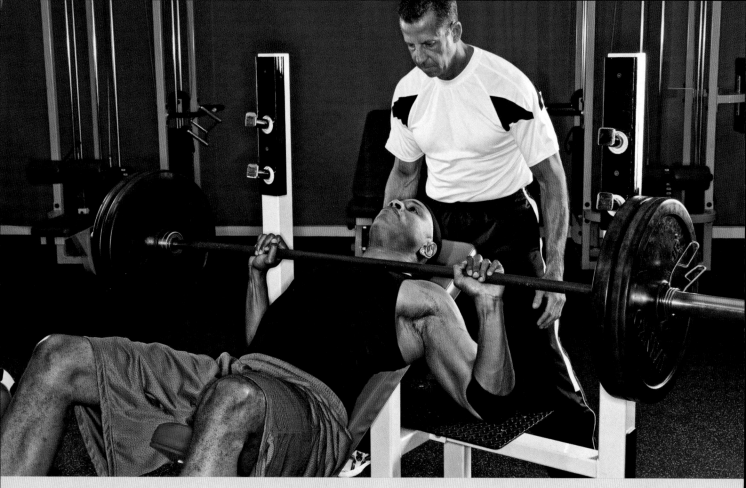

Incline Bench Press: Lie on an incline bench set at approximately 30 to 45 degrees. Spread your legs slightly with your feet flat on the floor. Grasp the barbell with a pronated (overhand) grip with a wider than shoulder-width grip. Unrack the bar and hold it directly above your upper chest. Slowly lower the bar to your upper chest. Without bouncing the bar off your chest, powerfully press the bar back up to the start position. Pause momentarily in the top position before repeating for reps.

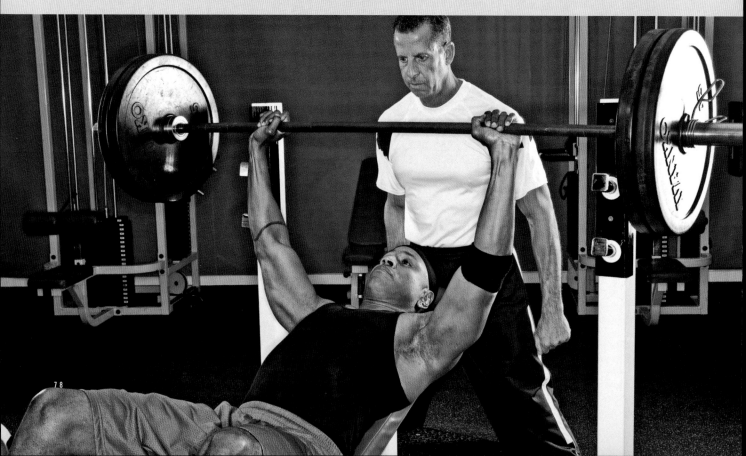

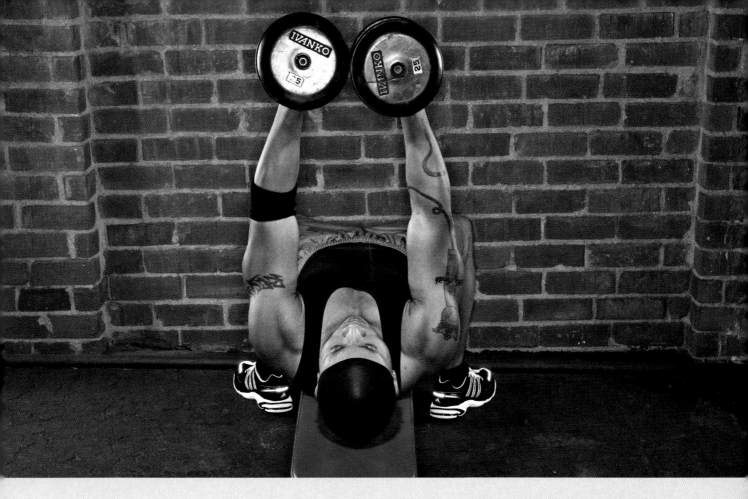

Flat-Bench Dumbbell Fly: Lie faceup on the bench with your feet flat on the floor. Hold a dumbbell in each hand with a neutral grip and extend your arms above your chest. Slowly lower the dumbbells in a wide arc down to your sides, keeping your elbows locked in a slightly bent position throughout the range of motion. Stop when your elbows reach shoulder level and reverse the motion.

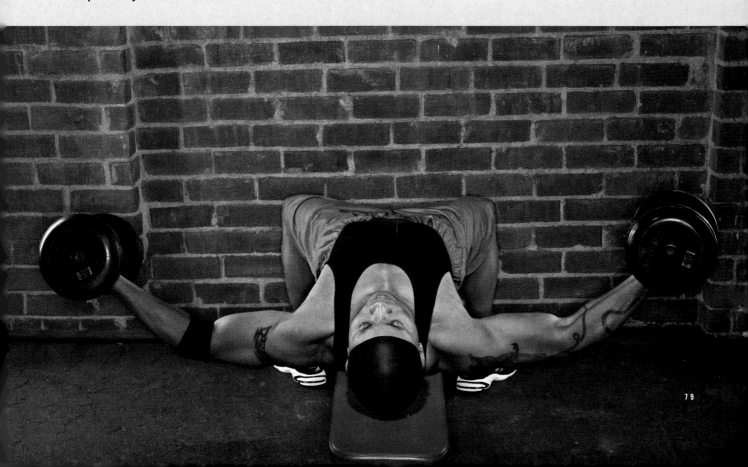

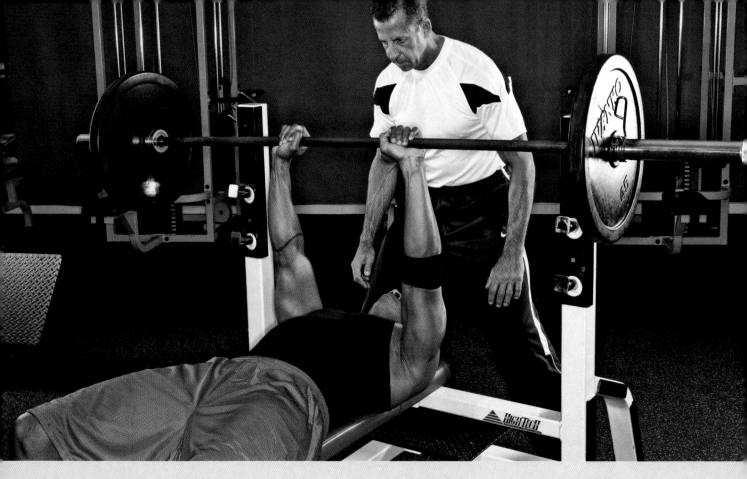

Close-Grip Bench Press: Lie faceup on a bench with your feet flat on the floor. Grasp the barbell with an overhand grip, your hands about 12 inches apart. Unrack the bar and slowly lower it toward your chest. Keep your elbows pointed out to your sides. When the bar just touches your chest, press back up explosively, driving the weight away from you until you almost lock it out.

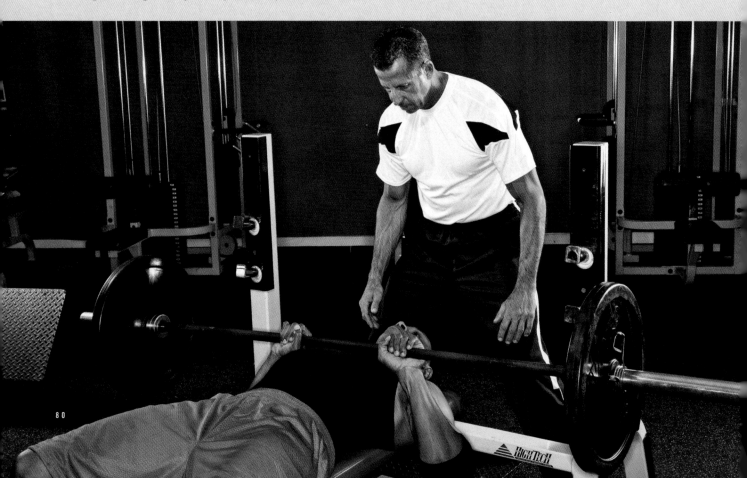

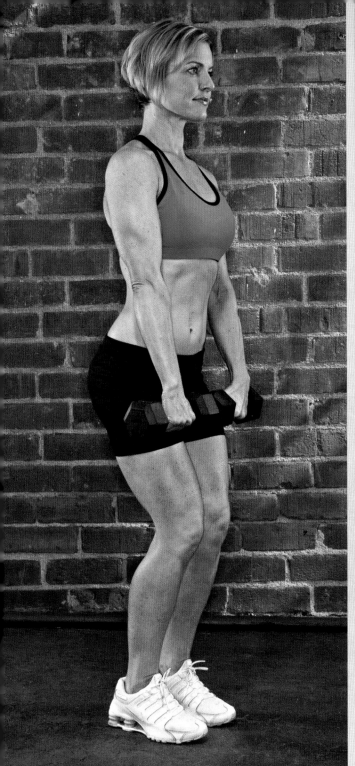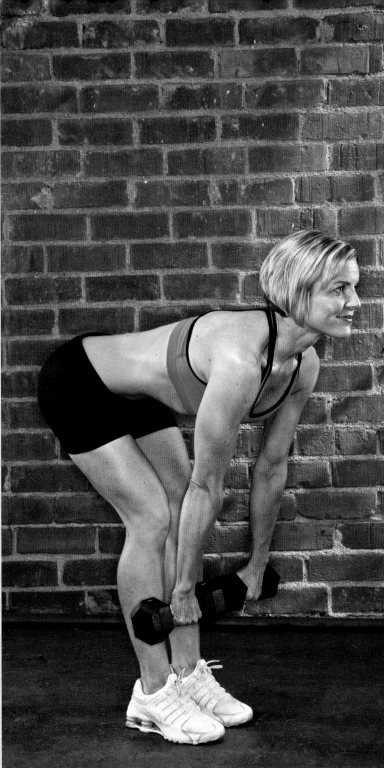

Romanian Deadlift: Stand upright holding dumbbells or a barbell in front of your upper thighs with a pronated (overhand) grip. Keep your feet shoulder-width apart and a slight bend in your knees. Keeping your chest up, abs tight, and the natural arch in your low back, lean forward from your hips, pushing them rearward until your torso is roughly parallel to the floor. As you lean forward, keep your arms straight and slide the dumbbells or bar down your thighs toward the floor until the weight reaches your shins. At the bottom, keep your back flat and head neutral, with the dumbbells or bar very close to your legs. From there, flex your hamstrings and glutes and lift your torso while pushing your hips forward until you return to the start position.

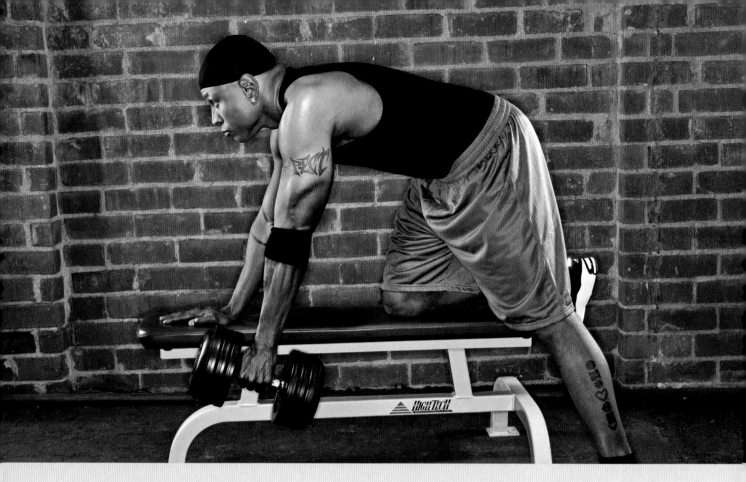

Dumbbell Row: Place one knee and the same-side hand on a flat bench, with your other foot on the floor beside the bench. Hold a dumbbell in your free hand, hanging it straight down with your arm fully extended. Pull the weight toward your hip, keeping your elbow in close and squeezing your shoulder blades together for a full contraction. Then lower the dumbbell along the same path. Repeat for reps, then switch arms.

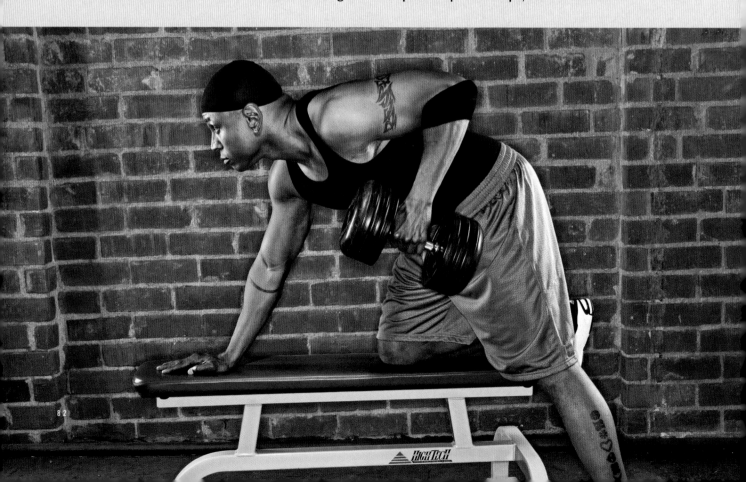

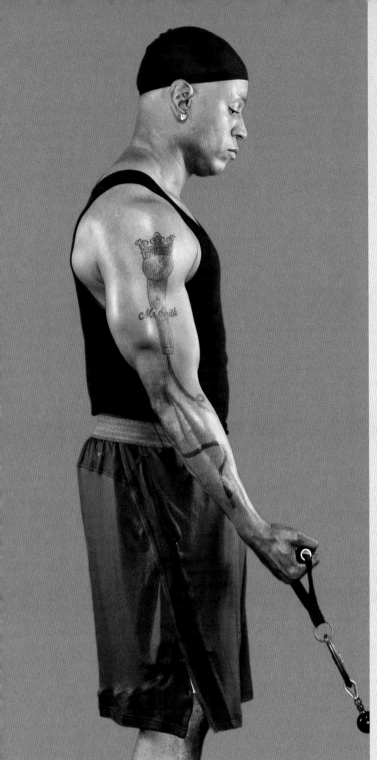
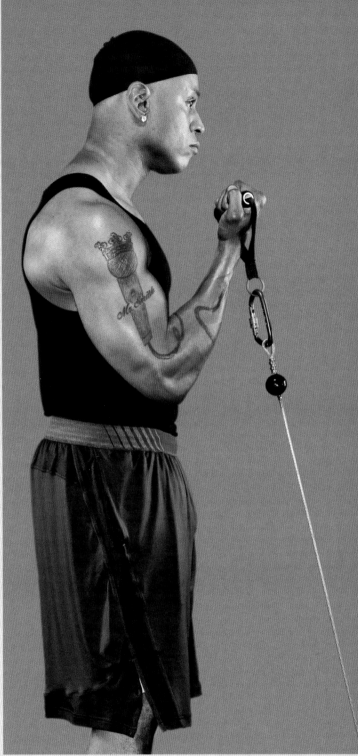

One-Arm Cable Curl: Stand in front of a low pulley cable. Bend over and grasp a D-handle with an underhand grip, locking your working arm against your same-side inner thigh, letting the cable travel under your leg. Place your nonworking arm on the same-side leg for balance. Moving only at your elbow, curl the handle as high as you can, squeeze your biceps at the top, then lower the cable back to the start without letting the weight stack touch down between reps.

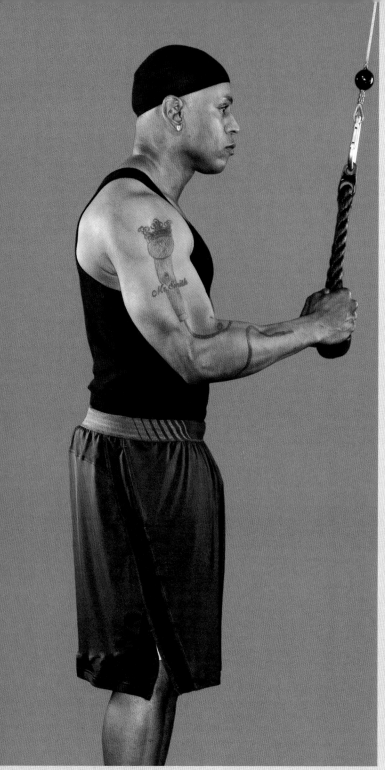
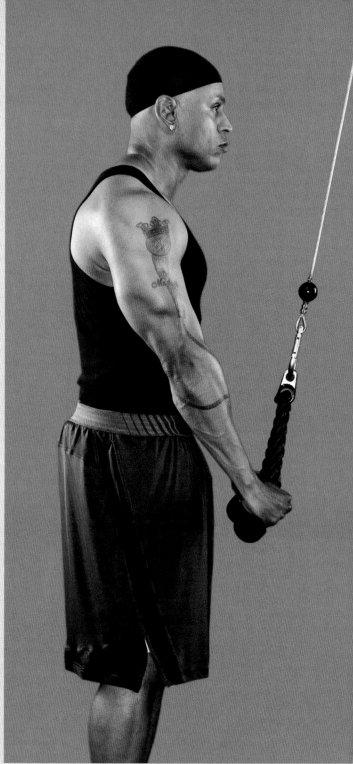

Rope Pressdown: Stand in front of a high cable pulley and grasp the rope attachment with a palms-facing-each-other grip. With your legs slightly bent, lean forward slightly at the waist and position your elbows close to your sides, your lower arms parallel to the floor. Press the bar down toward the floor until your arms are fully extended, pronating your hands at the bottom, hold for a brief count, and return to the start position.

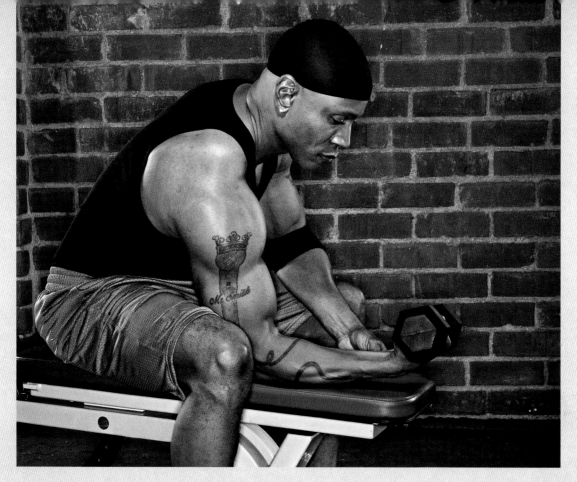

Dumbbell Wrist Curl: Sit at the end of a bench with your forearm flat on the bench and hold a dumbbell in your hand. Allow the dumbbell to roll to your fingers, then use your wrist to curl it back to the start. Finish all reps with one arm before switching.

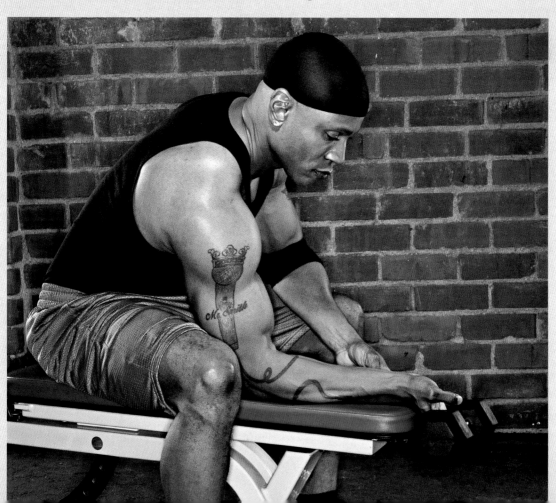

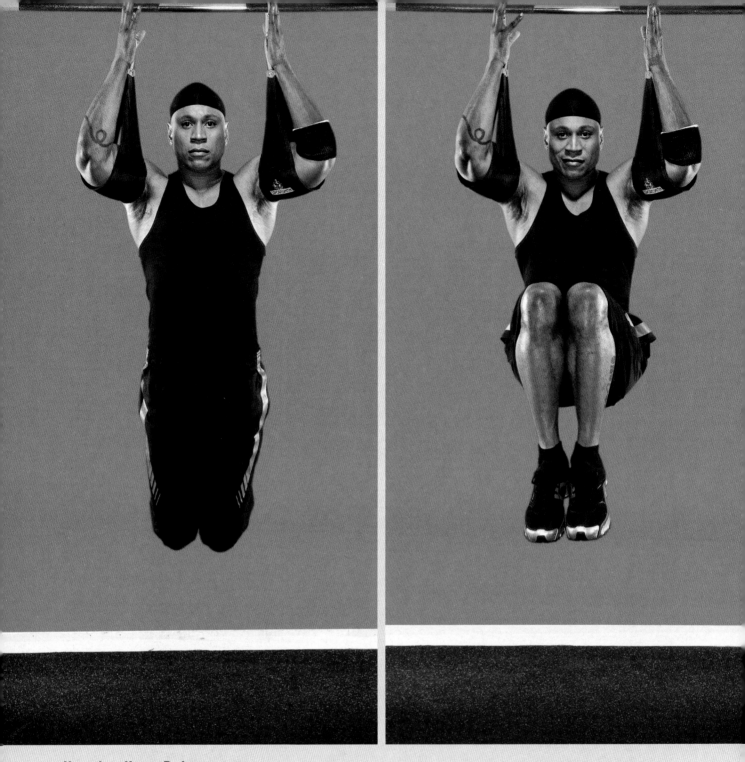

Hanging Knee Raise: Hanging from an overhead bar, contract your abs to bring your knees as high as possible in front of you. Pause and squeeze momentarily, then slowly lower your legs to the start position and repeat.

Scooter's Tip

Stretching before activity has become common for so-called "injury prevention," but it's not necessary. In fact, research has now made it clear that just as many people injure themselves if they stretch before weight training as those who don't. Add to that the fact that studies show stretching target muscles prior to a training session actually weakens them, hindering their performance and hurting your workouts. Instead, your best bet to start a weight workout is a gentle warmup, thoroughly saturating the muscles with blood with two to four very light weight, 15- to 30-rep sets of the first exercise.

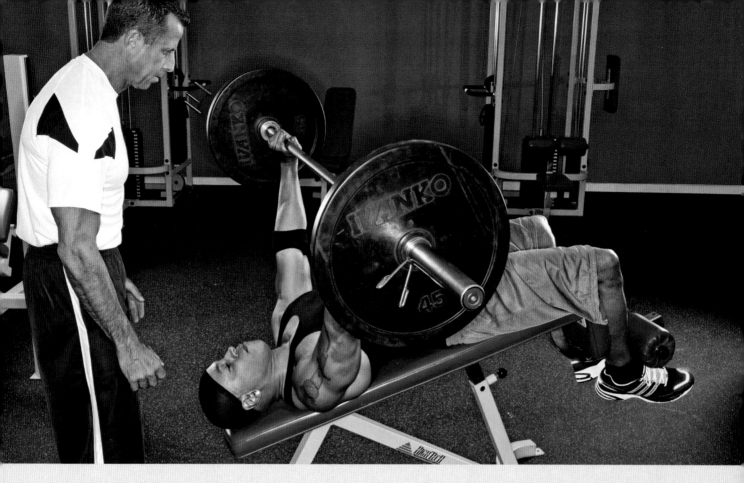

Decline Bench Press: Lie faceup on a decline bench adjusted to a 30-degree angle. Your torso should be fully supported from your head to your hips, with your knees bent and feet supported. Grasp the bar with a wide, overhand grip, unrack it, and hold it directly above you. Bend your arms and slowly lower the bar toward your lower chest. When the bar reaches chest level, forcefully extend your arms, pressing it back to the start position.

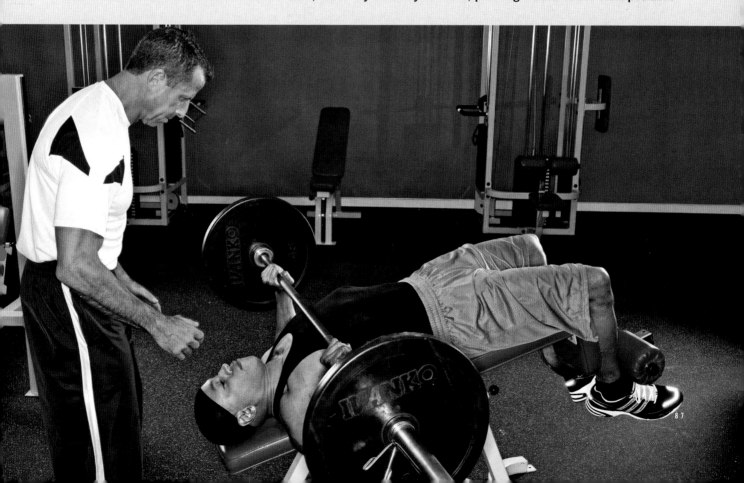

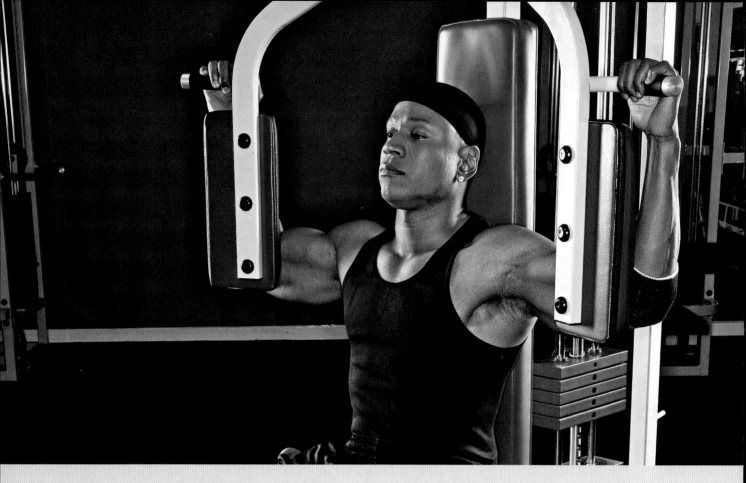

Pec-Deck Fly: Sit in the machine with your lower back fully supported and your feet flat on the floor. With your arms at 90-degree angles, place your lower arms flush against the pads and grasp the handles. Using your elbows, bring the handles together in front of your face, squeezing your chest hard, then slowly return to the start position, stopping when your upper arms are perpendicular to your torso.

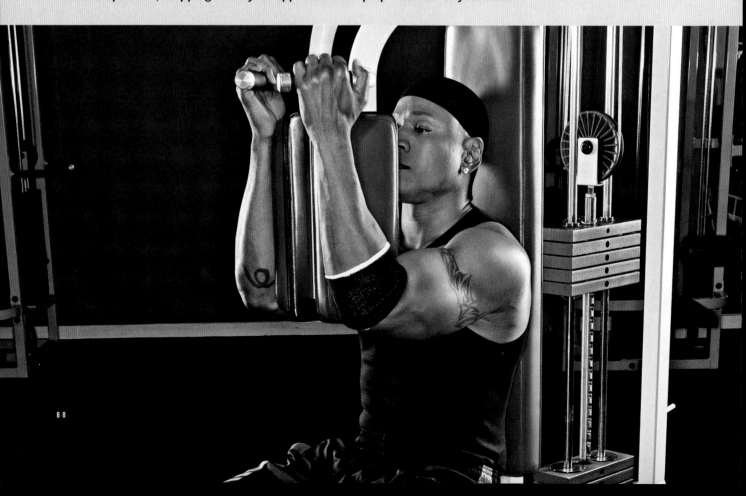

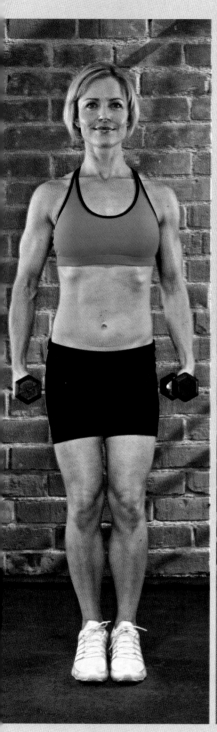
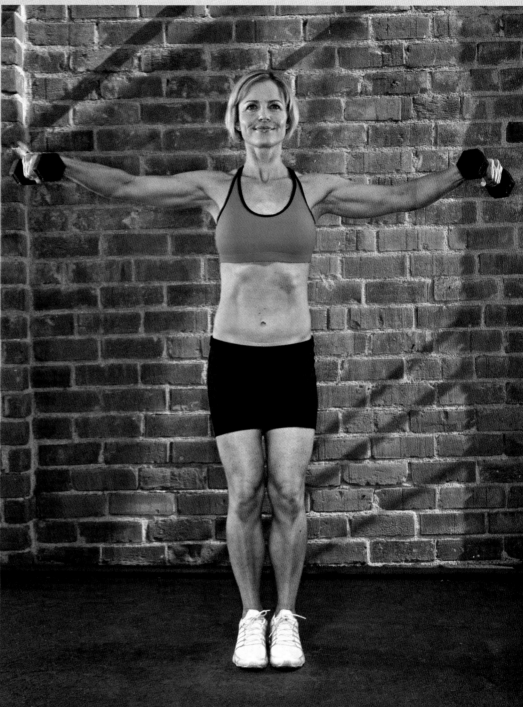

Dumbbell Lateral Raise: Stand with your feet together and your head straight, holding dumbbells at your sides with a neutral grip. Raise the dumbbells out to your sides in a wide arc, keeping your elbows and hands moving together in the same plane, to just above shoulder level. Hold momentarily in the peak contracted position, then slowly lower the dumbbells down along the same path.

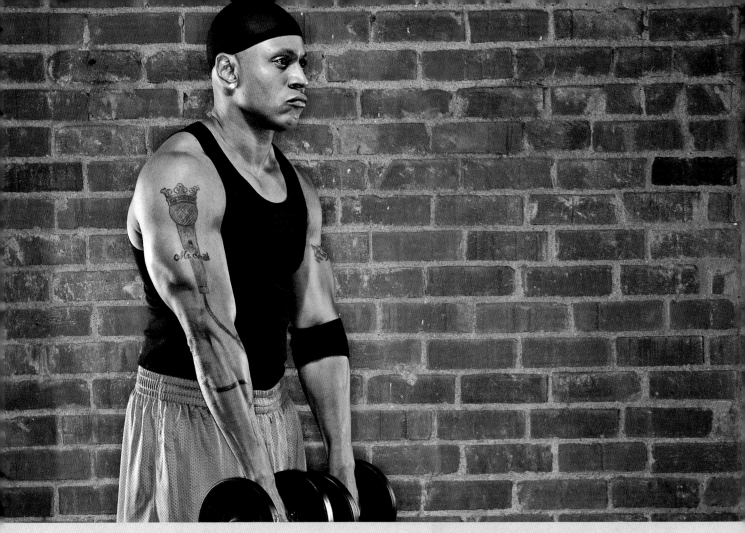

Dumbbell Front Raise: Stand holding a dumbbell in each hand directly in front of your thighs, your abs tight and chest up. Keeping your arms straight, raise the dumbbells in front of you just above parallel to the floor. Pause, then lower to the start position.

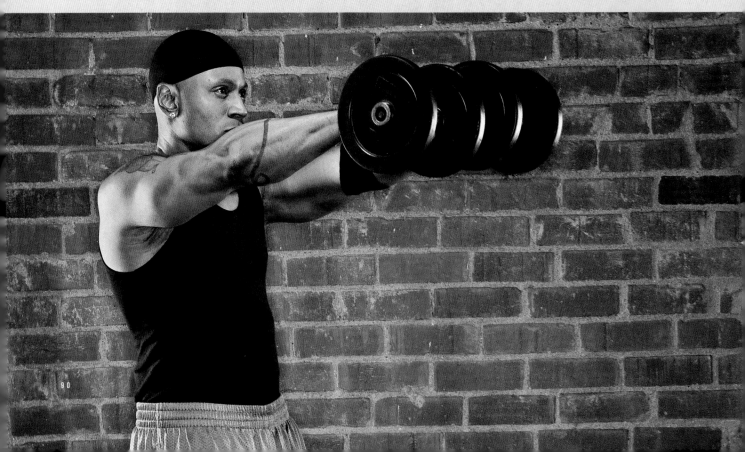

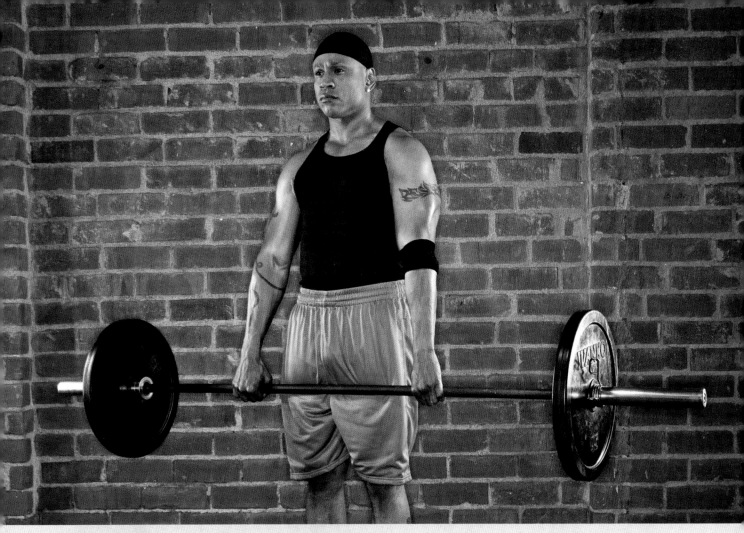

Barbell Shrug: Stand holding a barbell directly in front of your quads. With your chest up and abs tight, shrug your shoulders straight up toward the ceiling, squeezing your traps at the top. Slowly reverse the motion to lower back to the start position.

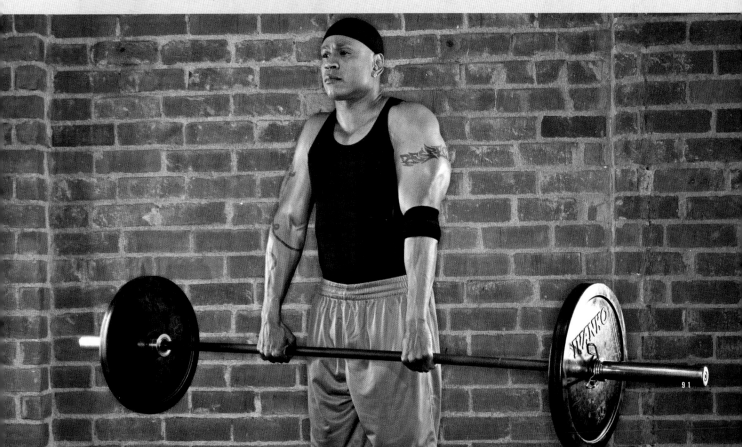

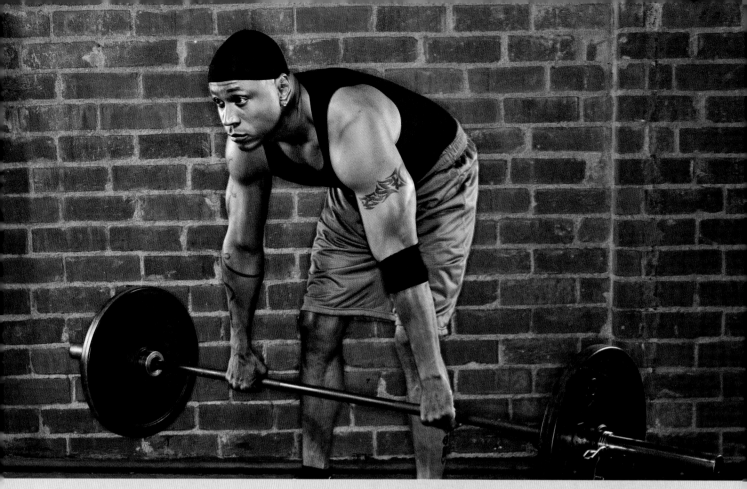

Bent-Over Barbell Row: Standing with your feet shoulder-width apart and knees slightly bent, grasp a barbell with a wide, overhand grip. Lean forward at your waist until your torso is roughly parallel to the floor. The barbell should hang straight down in front of your shins. Without raising your upper body, pull the barbell up toward your abdomen, bringing your elbows high and above the level of your back. Hold the bar in the peak contracted position for a brief count, then slowly lower along the same path.

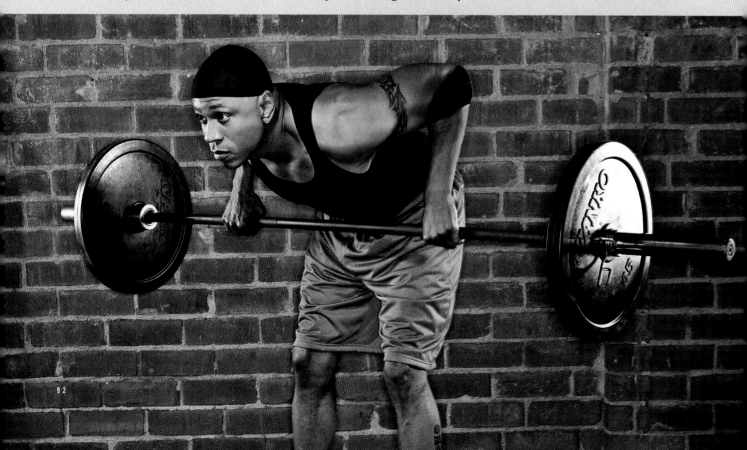

Scooter's Tip ▬

Don't worry about how much weight you're lifting.
Just make sure you're as intense and safe as possible.

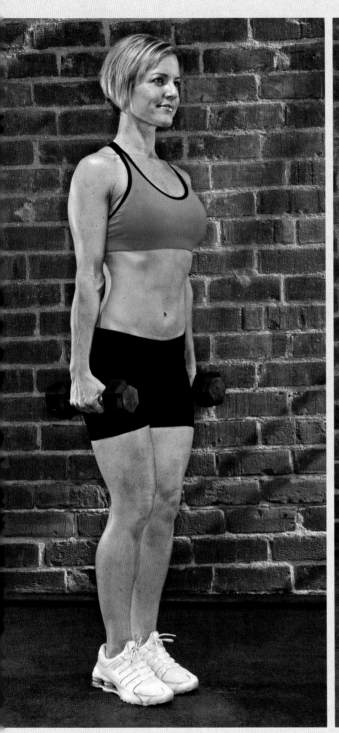
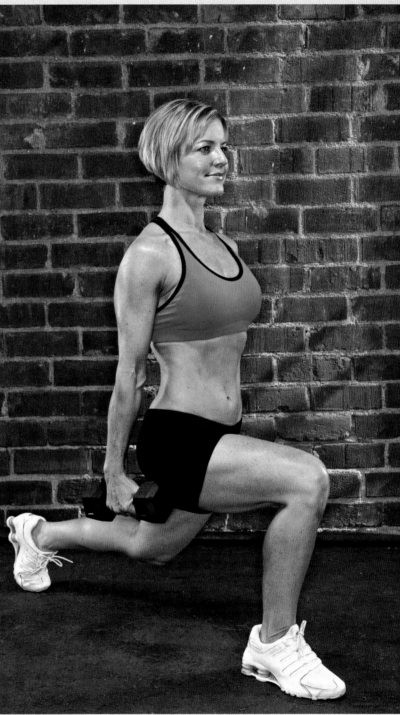

Walking Lunge: Holding a dumbbell in each hand, step forward with one foot. Bend both knees to lower yourself, making sure your front knee doesn't extend past your toes. Stop just short of your rear knee touching the floor and drive through the heel of your forward foot to bring your back leg forward to the front. Continue stepping deeply, moving across the gym—1 step with each foot equals 1 rep.

SCOOTER ON STRETCHING

You may think it's smart to start every workout with a few minutes of stretching, but here's something not many people understand: Stretching doesn't prevent injury. In fact, research shows that there are just as many injuries in people who do stretch before working out as there are in those who don't. What stretching can do is promote blood flow at the end of a training session (thus aiding recovery) and help minimize the effects of delayed-onset muscle soreness. That's why stretching—about 10 minutes' worth or so—is best done after your workout, when your muscles are warmed up and more pliable. Don't stretch cold.

If you find you lack the range of motion necessary to perform a specific exercise or move, do a couple of lightweight sets of the exercise you're attempting, then stretch the muscles gently and perform another warmup set. The more blood and water that flow to your muscles, the easier it will be to achieve the range of motion necessary to perform the exercise successfully and as safely as possible.

Here is a simple set of stretches to perform after your workout. Repeat each stretch two or three times, holding the stretch for about 15 seconds. Stretch only to the point of mild discomfort.

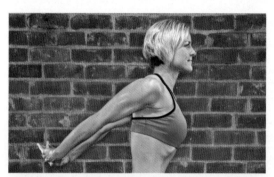

Chest and Biceps Stretch
Standing tall with your knees slightly bent, reach behind your back and clasp your hands together. Fully extend your elbows until your arms are straight, then elevate your arms until you feel the stretch.

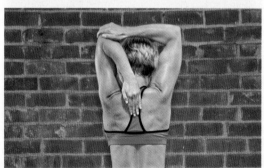

Single Arm Triceps and Lat Stretch
Standing tall, raise your arm straight up beside your head, then flex your elbow, reaching your hand toward the middle of your upper back. Use the opposite arm to gently pull your elbow inward, sliding your hand down your back until you feel the stretch. Repeat with your other arm.

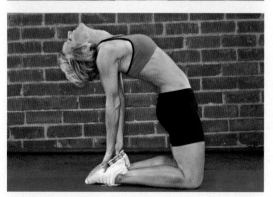

Kneeling Quadriceps Stretch
Kneeling on the floor, hold a heel in each hand. Lift your buttocks up by extending your hips forward and slightly arching your lower back. Tuck your toes for a more intense stretch.

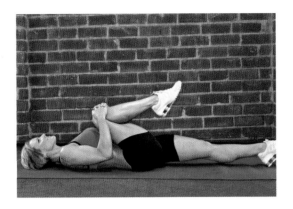

Lying Single Knee to the Chest Stretch

Lying on your back with both legs extended, lift your right leg, pulling your knee and thigh toward your chest. Keeping the left leg extended, gently apply pressure to the back of your right thigh until you feel the stretch. Repeat with the other leg.

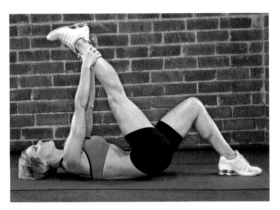

Lying Hamstring Stretch

Lying flat on your back, bend one knee, putting that foot flat on the floor to stabilize your core while your other leg remains extended. Raise your extended leg in the air and slightly bend the knee so that the sole of your foot faces the ceiling, then grasp your lower leg with your hands. Slowly straighten your legs as much as possible while gently pulling your extended leg toward your face. Repeat with your other leg.

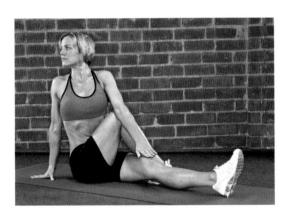

Lower Back Stretch

Sit on the floor with your legs extended out in front of your body and pull your right knee toward your chest. Cross it over your extended left leg so that your right foot is just beside your left knee. Place your left elbow against the outside of your right knee, extending your right arm slightly behind you to hold yourself upright. Slowly turn to the right until you feel the stretch. Repeat on the opposite side.

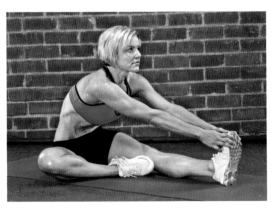

Modified Hurdler's Stretch

Sit on the floor with your left leg extended. Flex your right leg, pressing the sole of your foot against your left inner thigh. Keeping your back flat, lean forward at the hips, reaching for your toes until you feel the stretch. Flex your extended foot for a more intense stretch. Repeat with the opposite leg.

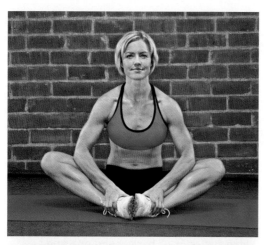

Butterfly

Sit on the floor with your legs bent and the soles of your feet pressed together. Keeping your torso upright, lean forward at the hips, grasp your feet, and place your elbows against your inner thighs. Gently apply pressure with your elbows and pull yourself forward, keeping your back flat, until you feel the stretch.

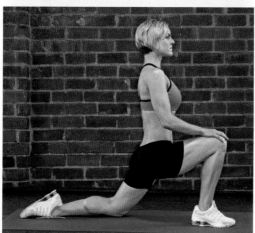

Kneeling Hip Flexor Stretch

Kneel on a mat with one knee on the floor and the other flexed at a 90-degree angle. Shift your weight forward until you feel a mild stretch in your hip. Repeat on the other side.

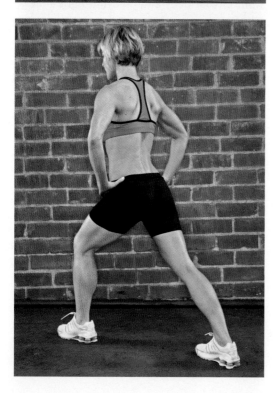

Standing Calf Stretch

Stand with your feet shoulder-width apart. Extend one leg behind you, keeping both feet flat on the floor. Lean forward until you feel the stretch in the extended calf. Repeat with the other leg.

THE PLATINUM 360 WORKOUT RECAP

Note: All workouts list exercise, number of sets, and total reps per set.

PHASE 1: Weeks 1 and 2

Do this workout three times per week on nonconsecutive days (such as Monday, Wednesday, and Friday).

Leg Press	2 x 12–15
Leg Extension	2 x 12–15
Lying Leg Curl	2 x 12–15
Lat Pulldown	2 x 12–15
Machine Chest Press	2 x 12–15
Machine Row	2 x 12–15
Overhead Machine Press	2 x 12–15

Machine Preacher Curl	2 x 12–15
Cable Pressdown	2 x 12–15
Standing Calf Raise	2 x 12–15
Crunch	2 x 12–15

Rest 30 seconds between sets.

Cardio: Steady-state (slow and easy) cardio done for 20 minutes, three times per week, on a treadmill, stationary bike, step mill, or stairclimber or outdoors.

PHASE 2: Weeks 3 and 4

Do each of the following workouts twice this week; for instance, the upper-body session can be done on Monday and Thursday, while the lower-body workout can be completed on Tuesday and Friday.

Days 1 and 4: Upper Body

Smith Bench Press	3 x 8–12
Seated Cable Row	3 x 8–12
Standing Overhead Press	2 x 8–12
Barbell Curl	3 x 8–12
Cable Pressdown	3 x 8–12
Cable Crunch	3 x 8–12

Days 3, 6, and 7: Rest

Days 2 and 5: Lower Body

Smith Squat	3 x 8–12
Leg Press	3 x 8–12
Dumbbell Stepup	2 x 8–12
Leg Extension	3 x 8–12
Barbell Lunge	3 x 8–12
Lying Leg Curl	3 x 8–12
Seated Calf Raise	2 x 8–12

In both workouts, rest 1 minute between sets.

Cardio: Perform two 30-minute steady-state workouts (slow and easy) on Days 1 and 4 and two 20-minute interval cardio workouts on Days 2 and 5, for a total of four cardio sessions per week.

PHASE 3: Weeks 5 and 6

You'll do each of the following workouts twice this week.

Days 1 and 5: Chest, Shoulders, Triceps

Dumbbell Bench Press	3 x 8–12
Incline Cable Fly	3 x 8–12
Weighted Dip	2 x 8–12
Upright Row	3 x 8–12
Seated Overhead Dumbbell Press	3 x 8–12
Cable Lateral Raise	2 x 8–12
Cable Kickback	3 x 8–12
Reverse-Grip Pressdown	3 x 8–12
Bench Dip	2 x 8–12
Overhead Cable Extension	2 x 8–12

Days 2 and 6: Legs

Barbell Squat	3 x 8–12
Leg Press	3 x 8–12
Hack Squat	2 x 8–12
Leg Extension	3 x 8–12
Barbell Lunge	3 x 8–12
Lying Leg Curl	3 x 8–12
Standing Calf Raise	2 x 8–12
Seated Calf Raise	2 x 8–12

Days 3 and 7: Back, Biceps, Abs, Calves

Straight-Arm Pulldown	3 x 8–12
Dumbbell Pullover	3 x 8–12
T-Bar Row	2 x 8–12
Dumbbell Curl	3 x 8–12
Incline Dumbbell Curl	3 x 8–12
Dumbbell Preacher Curl	2 x 8–12
Hanging Leg Raise	3 x 8–12
Weighted Crunch	3 x 8–12
Standing Calf Raise	3 x 8–12

Rest 1 minute between all sets in all workouts.

Cardio: Perform two 35-minute interval cardio workouts with the chest, shoulders, and triceps sessions and two 25-minute steady-state cardio workouts with the leg sessions, for a total of four cardio workouts per week.

Day 4: Rest

PHASE 4: Weeks 7 and 8

You'll do each of the workouts once per week, making sure to never work out more than 2 days in a row without inserting a day of rest.

Day 1: Chest, Shoulders, Triceps, Abs

Incline Bench Press*	4 x 12, 12, 8, 8
Flat-Bench Dumbbell Fly	3 x 12, 10, 8
Bench Dip	3 x 12, 10, 8
Seated Overhead Dumbbell Press*	4 x 12, 12, 6, 6
Upright Row	3 x 8, 6, 6
Cable Lateral Raise	3 x 12, 12, 12
Close-Grip Bench Press	3 x 12, 12, 12
Rope Pressdown*	3 x 15, 10, 8
Cable Crunch	3 x to failure

superset with

Hanging Leg Raise	3 x to failure

Day 2: Legs, Calves, Back, Biceps, Forearms, Abs

Leg Press*	4 x 12, 12, 8, 6
Leg Extension	3 x 10, 10, 8
Lying Leg Curl	3 x 10, 10, 8
Romanian Deadlift	3 x 10, 10, 8
Seated Calf Raise	4 x 25, 25, 12, 12
Lat Pulldown*	3 x 12, 8, 8
Seated Cable Row (wide grip)	3 x 12, 12, 12
Dumbbell Row	3 x 12, 12, 12
Barbell Curl*	4 x 12, 10, 8, 6
Incline Dumbbell Curl	3 x 10, 10, 8
One-Arm Cable Curl	3 x 10, 10, 8
Dumbbell Wrist Curl*	3 x 12, 10, 10
Hanging Knee Raise	3 x to failure
Crunch	2 x 15, 15

Days 3, 5, and 7: Rest

Day 4: Chest, Shoulders, Traps, Triceps, Abs

Decline Bench Press*	3 x 12, 10, 8
Dumbbell Bench Press	3 x 10, 8, 6
Pec-Deck Fly	3 x 10, 8, 6
Overhead Machine Press*	4 x 12, 10, 8, 6
Dumbbell Lateral Raise	3 x 10, 8, 6
Dumbbell Front Raise	3 x 10, 10, 10
Barbell Shrug	3 x 6, 6, 6
Straight-Bar Cable Pressdown*	3 x 10, 10, 8
Overhead Cable Extension	3 x 10, 8, 6
Weighted Dip	3 x 10, 8, 6
Hanging Knee Raise	3 x to failure
Weighted Crunch	2 x to failure

Day 6: Legs, Back, Biceps, Abs

Smith Squat	4 x 10, 10, 6, 6
Walking Lunge	3 x 10, 10, 8
Lying Leg Curl	3 x 10, 10, 8
Romanian Deadlift	3 x 10, 10, 8
Standing Calf Raise*	3 x 10, 12, 15
Bent-Over Barbell Row	3 x 10, 8, 6
Seated Cable Row	3 x 10, 8, 6
Lat Pulldown	3 x 12, 12, 12
Dumbbell Curl*	4 x 10, 8, 6, 6
Dumbbell Preacher Curl	3 x 10, 8, 6
Crunch	3 x to failure
Hanging Leg Raise	3 x to failure

Perform as a drop set; the reps listed are the number you do before dropping the weight. On that first drop, continue until muscle failure. Rest 2 minutes between drop sets.

Cardio: You'll perform two 35-minute interval cardio workouts with the Day 1 and Day 4 sessions and two 25-minute steady-state cardio workouts with the Day 2 and Day 6 sessions, for a total of four cardio workouts per week. Do your cardio after your weight sessions for best results.

CHAPTER 5
SCOOTER'S ADVANCED PROGRAM AND 30-MINUTE WORKOUTS

If you've made it through the 8-Week Workout plan, congratulations are in order. But it's not the end of the road. Think of the Platinum 360 8-Week program as your undergraduate work, a great foundation for a leaner, fitter body that you will carry with you as you proceed on your journey. What you need now is some postgrad studies, the specialized lessons that will help you continue to set and reach new goals. That's where Scooter's Advanced Program and mini workouts come in. I like to think of the Advanced Program as the fifth phase of the 8-Week Workout—not exactly a maintenance plan, but rather a blueprint for going further, reaching higher. This is a truly tough workout, not something you will master in a week or maybe even a month—especially if you're adding weights and reps to the workout as you go—so if you want to switch back and forth between the Advanced Program and Phase 4 of the 8-Week plan, no problem. You might also want to ratchet up the intensity of your Week 4 workout by adding an extra mini workout from the 30-Minute section, putting extra focus on a particular part of the body. You can also use the 30-Minute routines on days when time is tight, or combine two or more for your own personalized workout. It's really a mix-and-match menu that will allow you to craft workouts that continually challenge you and keep things interesting.

THE ADVANCED PROGRAM

For this phase, you'll take the training split one more step, dividing your body into four distinct workouts. These sessions run the full spectrum of repetition ranges, from low reps—6 per set—that help elevate your metabolism during and hours after your workout to high reps—25 per set—that will flush your muscles with blood and nutrients for recovery.

There's another major addition in this workout: plyometric and cardio activity between sets. Plyometrics—which are explosive movements that engage your body's myostatic reflex via the quick stretch and engage your fast-twitch muscle fibers to ultimately generate power—are a valuable partner to traditional weight training. The activities include traditional jumping rope, jump squats (where you go down into a squat position and jump up as high as you can), split jump squats (where you do jump squats from a staggered stance), and lateral box jumps (where you jump side to side over a 2- to 3-foot-high box or platform).

For cardio, you'll do both steady and interval cardio, with longer steady-pace sessions to challenge your cardiovascular system and burn off extra calories.

PHASE 5 TRAINING SPLIT

DAY	MODE
1	Arms
2	Legs
3	Cardio, abs
4	Chest, shoulders
5	Back, traps
6	Cardio, abs, calves
7	Rest

THE PLATINUM 360 ADVANCED WORKOUTS

You'll do each of the following workouts once per week, as laid out below and on the next pages.

Day 1: Arms

Exercise	Sets	Reps	Time
Barbell Curl (page 49)	3	6, 8, 25	
Jump Rope			1 minute
Preacher Curl	3	6, 8, 25	
Jump Squat			1 minute
Incline Cable Curl	3	6, 8, 25	
Jump Rope			1 minute
Lying Triceps Extension	3	6, 8, 25	
Jump Squat			1 minute
Rope Pressdown (page 84)	3	6, 8, 25	
Jump Rope			1 minute
Overhead Dumbbell Extension	3	6, 8, 25	
Jump Squat			1 minute

Day 2: Legs

Exercise	Sets	Reps	Time
Barbell Squat (page 67)	3	6, 8, 25	
Lateral Box Hops			1 minute
Hack Squat (page 67)	3	6, 8, 25	
Split-Jump Squat			1 minute
Leg Extension (page 34)	3	6, 8, 25	
Lateral Box Hops			1 minute
Romanian Deadlift (page 81)	3	6, 8, 25	
Split-Jump Squat			1 minute
Seated Leg Curl	3	6, 8, 25	
Lateral Box Hops			1 minute
Standing Calf Raise (page 42)	3	6, 8, 25	
Split-Jump Squat			1 minute
Seated Calf Raise (page 54)	3	6, 8, 25	
Lateral Box Hops			1 minute

*Rest 1 minute between sets. Once you've completed all 3 sets of an exercise, perform 1 minute of activity, as indicated.

Day 3: Cardio and Abs

Exercise	Sets	Reps
Hanging Knee Raise (page 86)	3	To failure
Crunch (page 43)	3	To failure
Knee-Ins	3	To failure
Standing Calf Raise (page 42)	3	To failure
Seated Calf Raise (page 54)	3	To failure

Cardio: Start workout with a bout on the treadmill, stairclimber, or step mill for 1 full hour.

Day 4: Chest, Shoulders

Exercise	Sets	Reps	Time
Incline Bench Press (page 78)	3	6, 8, 25	
Jump Rope			1 minute
Incline Cable Fly (page 58)	3	6, 8, 25	
Jump Squat			1 minute
Smith Bench Press (page 46)	3	6, 8, 25	
Jump Rope			1 minute
Incline-Bench Cable Fly	3	6, 8, 25	
Jump Squat			1 minute
Decline Press	3	6, 8, 25	
Jump Rope			1 minute
Standing Overhead Press (page 48)	3	6, 8, 25	
Jump Squat			1 minute
Cable Lateral Raise (page 62)	3	6, 8, 25	
Jump Rope			1 minute
Bent-Over Cable Lateral Raise	3	6, 8, 25	
Jump Squat			1 minute

Day 5: Back, Traps

Exercise	Sets	Reps	Time
Deadlift	3	6, 8, 25	
Lateral Box Hops			1 minute
Dumbbell Row (page 82)	3	6, 8, 25	
Split-Jump Squat			1 minute
Reverse-Grip Lat Pulldown	3	6, 8, 25	
Lateral Box Hops			1 minute
Seated Cable Row (wide grip) (page 47)	3	6, 8, 25	
Split-Jump Squat			1 minute
Barbell Shrug (page 91)	3	6, 8, 25	
Lateral Box Hops			1 minute
Dumbbell Shrug	3	6, 8, 25	
Split-Jump Squat			1 minute
Pullup	3	To failure	

*Rest 1 minute between sets. Once you've completed all 3 sets of an exercise, perform 1 minute of activity, as indicated.

Day 6: Cardio, Abs, Calves

Exercise	Sets	Reps
Hanging Knee Raise (page 86)	3	To failure
Machine Crunch	3	10–12
Standing Calf Raise (page 42)	3	20
Seated Calf Raise (page 54)	3	20

* Rest 1 minute between sets in all workouts.

Cardio: Precede abs and calves with a 1-hour session on the treadmill or stairclimber at a steady pace.

EXERCISE INSTRUCTIONS

Note: All new exercises introduced in the Advanced Program are on the following pages; the other descriptions can be found in Phases 1 through 4, as they carry over.

Scooter's Tip
You need to frame how you respond to challenges. There is no "I'll try"—there is only "I'll do."

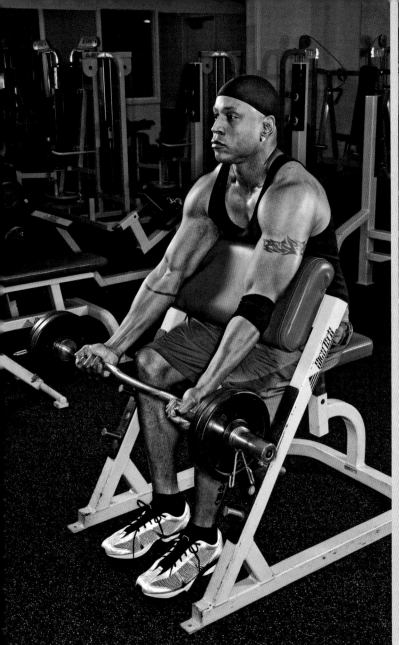
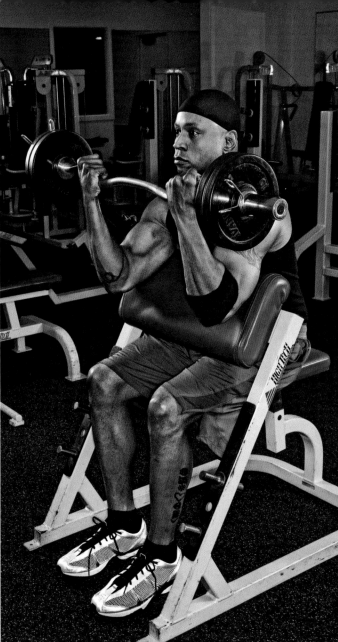

Preacher Curl: Set up a preacher bench so that the top of the pad fits securely under your armpits. Take a shoulder-width, underhand grip on the bar and position your arms parallel to each other on the bench. Keep your feet flat on the floor and your head straight. Flex your biceps to bring the bar as high as possible without allowing your elbows to flare out, squeeze hard at the top, and then slowly return the bar to the start position. Stop just short of full-arm extension and repeat for reps.

Scooter's Tip

As you advance through this program, we throw things at you like supersets and drop sets and other intensity techniques. These are ways to make a standard exercise harder—and harder can be better when it comes to lifting. For your muscles to respond and grow, you need to break them down. You need to push them further than they are used to going and literally force them to grow. If they aren't challenged, what impetus do they have to get bigger and stronger?

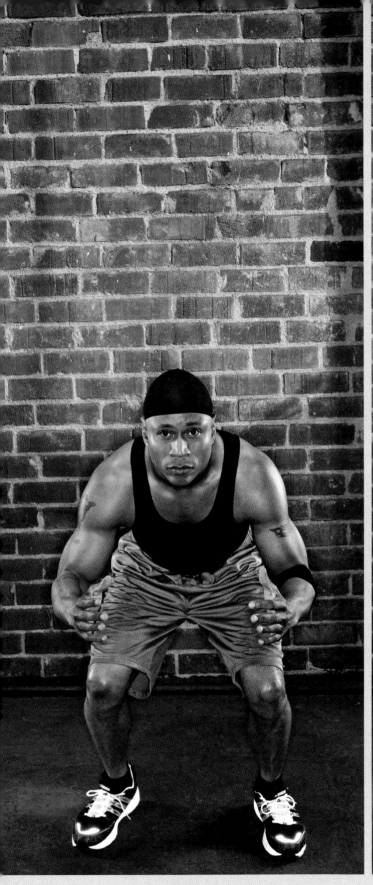
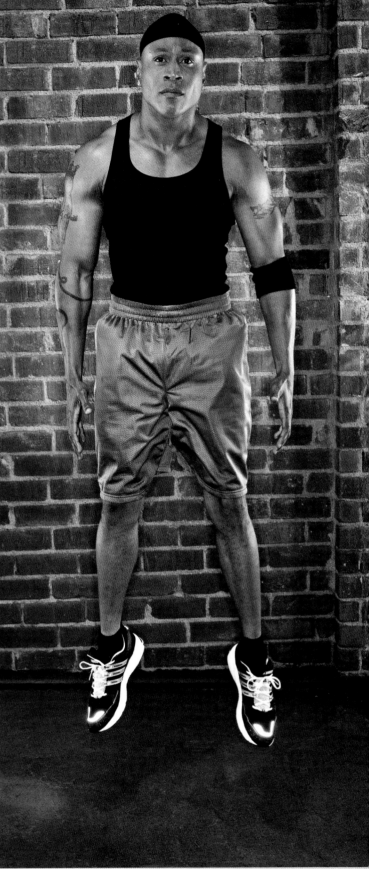

Jump Squat: Stand with both hands directly in front of you, knees slightly bent in roughly a shoulder-width stance. Keeping your chest up and back flat, squat down until your thighs approach parallel to the floor, then explode upward as high as possible, allowing your feet to leave the floor. Land on soft feet with your knees bent and repeat immediately.

THE PLATINUM 360 FITNESS PLAN

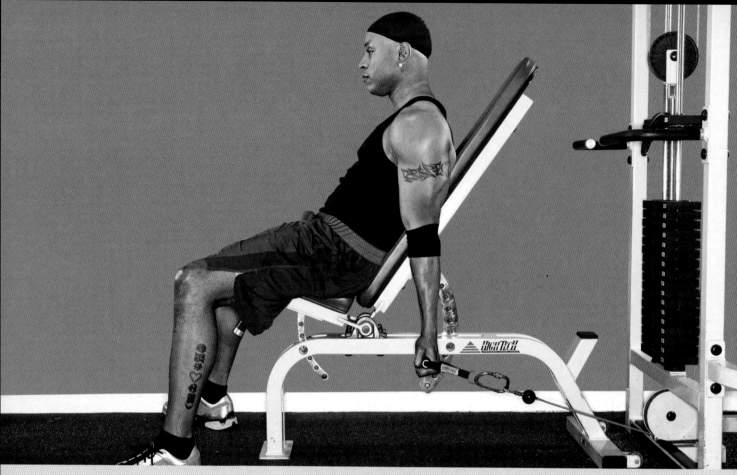

Incline Cable Curl: Place an incline bench adjusted to about 45 to 60 degrees, facing out from a cable stack with a D-handle attached to the lower pulley. Sit back squarely against the bench, feet flat on the floor. Your working arm should hang straight down by your side, palms up, holding the handle. Keeping your shoulders back and upper arms in a fixed position perpendicular to the floor, curl the handle so it approaches your shoulders. Squeeze your biceps hard at the top before slowly returning to the start position. Finish all reps with one side, then switch to the other arm.

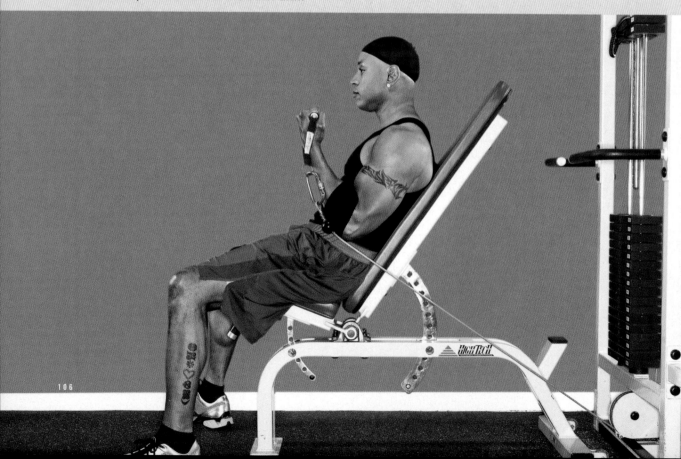

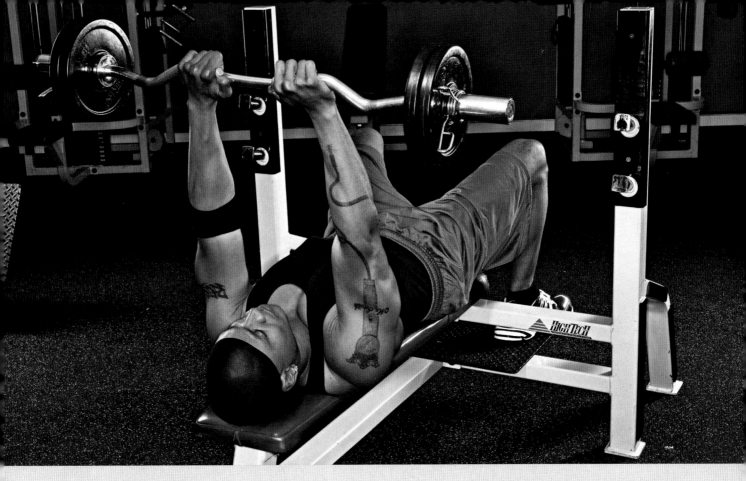

Lying Triceps Extension: Lie faceup on a flat bench with your feet flat on the floor, and have a partner hand you a straight bar (or EZ-bar) and grasp it with an overhand grip. With your arms extended, hold the bar at a 45-degree angle above your head, back toward your spotter. Slowly lower the bar down toward the top of your head. When you reach a 90-degree angle in your elbows, pause for a moment, then forcefully extend your arms and return the bar to the start position.

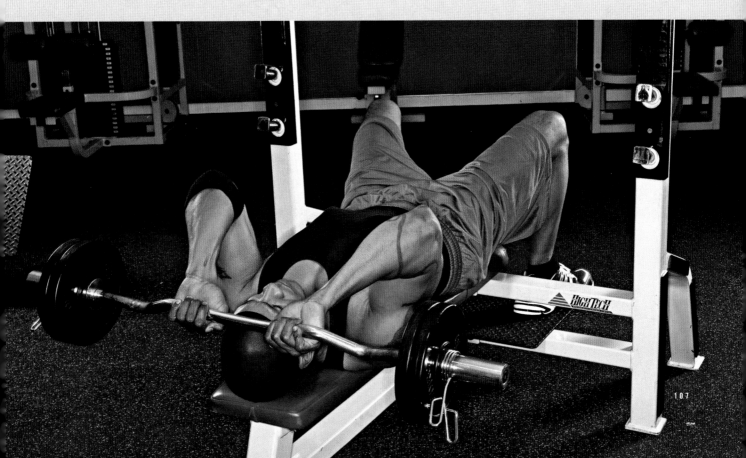

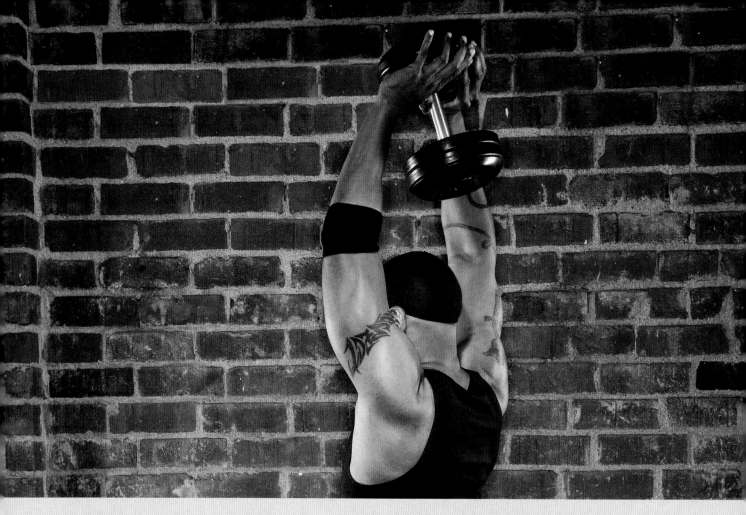

Overhead Dumbbell Extension: Stand holding a dumbbell with both hands, hand-over-hand style, with your arms extended overhead. Keep your abs tight, eyes forward, back straight, and upper arms next to your ears. Moving only your lower arms, bend your elbows to lower the weight behind your head, squeeze your triceps hard, and return to the start position.

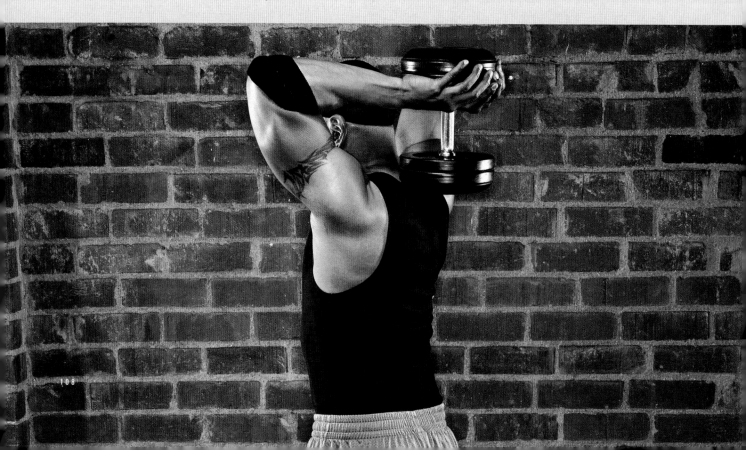

Scooter's Tip
If you want to get somewhere, you need to stretch yourself.
Do things that aren't easy. Don't avoid the hard exercises.

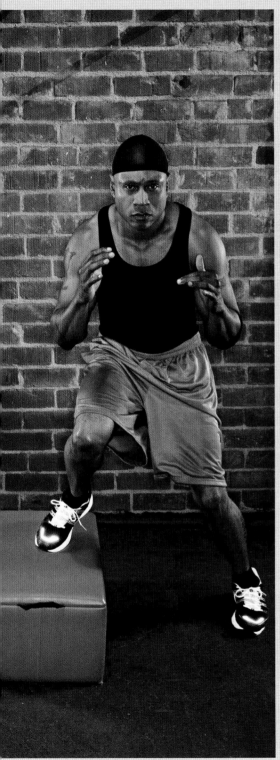
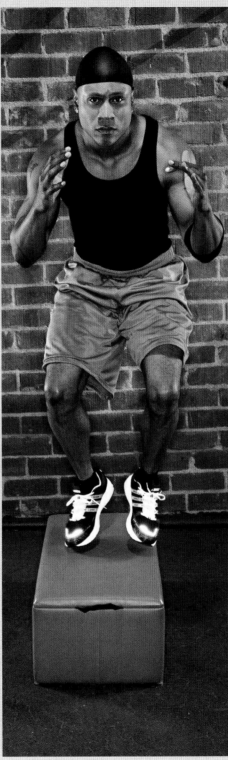
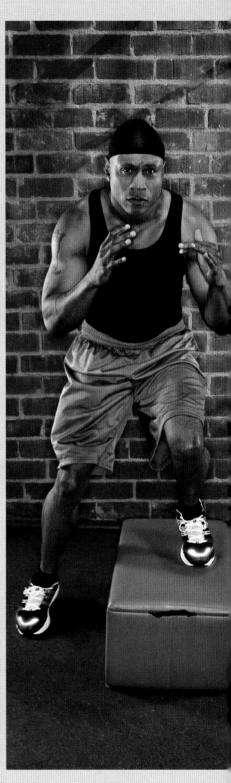

Lateral Box Hops: Stand sideways, feet together, next to an elevated platform like a box (advanced athletes can use a sturdy flat bench). From that position, leap upward onto the box or bench, land softly, and then leap again to the other side. Continue back and forth over the box/bench in that pattern.

Scooter's Tip

Unless it's the primary focus of your training, do cardio after, not before, you lift weights. You want to be at your strongest when you're lifting weight, and blowing all of your energy on cardio will just leave you depleted and struggling. The more weight you can move with good form, the faster you'll see real results.

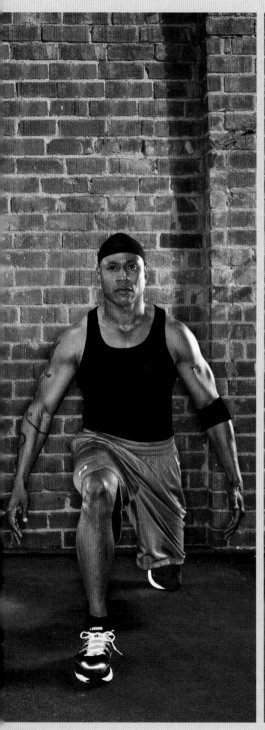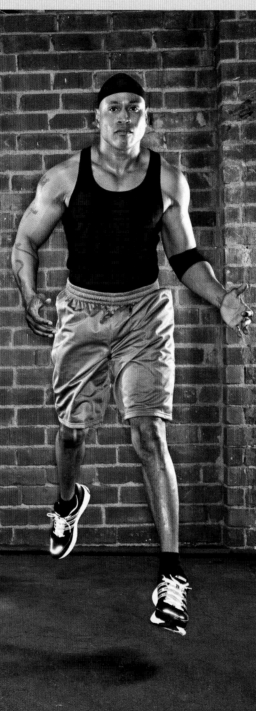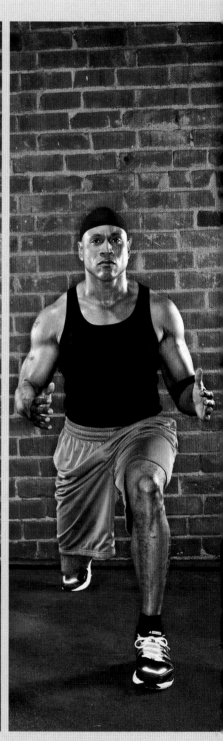

Split-Jump Squat: Step forward with one leg, as you would during a lunge. Keeping your chest up and back flat, bend both knees, lowering yourself toward the floor, then explode upward as high as possible, switching front and back legs in the air. Land on soft feet with your knees bent and repeat immediately.

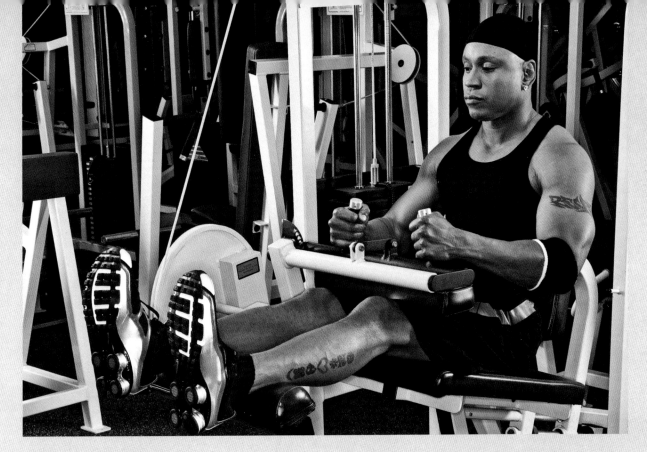

Seated Leg Curl: Sit in a leg-curl machine and position your Achilles tendons below the padded lever, your knees just off the edge of the bench, making sure the stability pad fits snugly over your lower thighs. Grasp the bench or the handles for stability. Make sure your knees are slightly bent to protect them from overextension. Bend your knees so your feet move toward your glutes in a strong but deliberate motion, squeezing the muscles at the bottom, then reverse to the start position without letting the weight stack touch down before beginning the next rep.

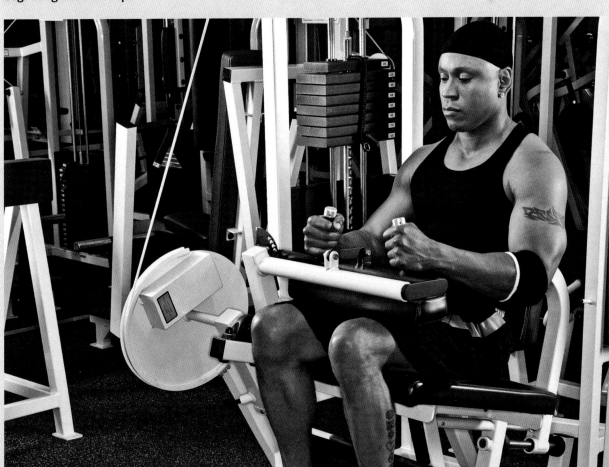

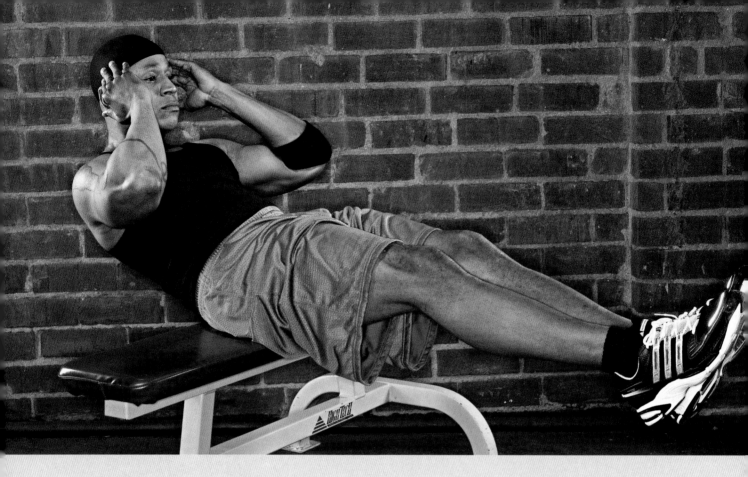

Knee-Ins: Sit on a bench with your hands cupped gently behind your head and your legs almost completely straight and raised a few inches. Simultaneously bring your knees to your torso while crunching your upper body toward your legs. Squeeze in the middle, then return to the start position and repeat. Don't let your feet go below parallel between reps.

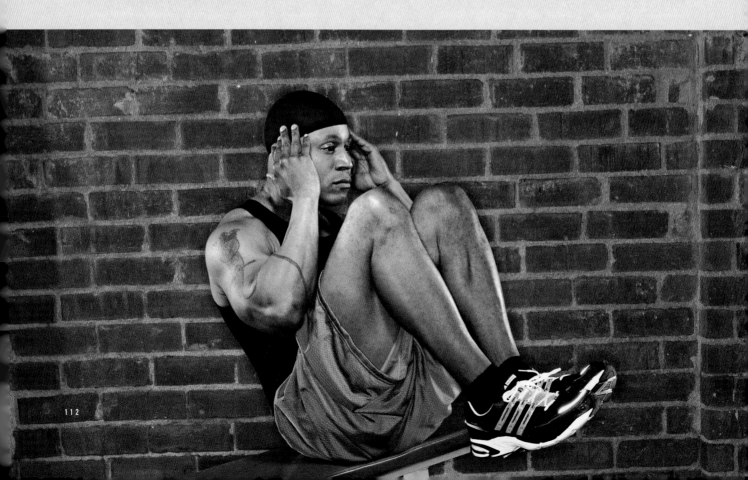

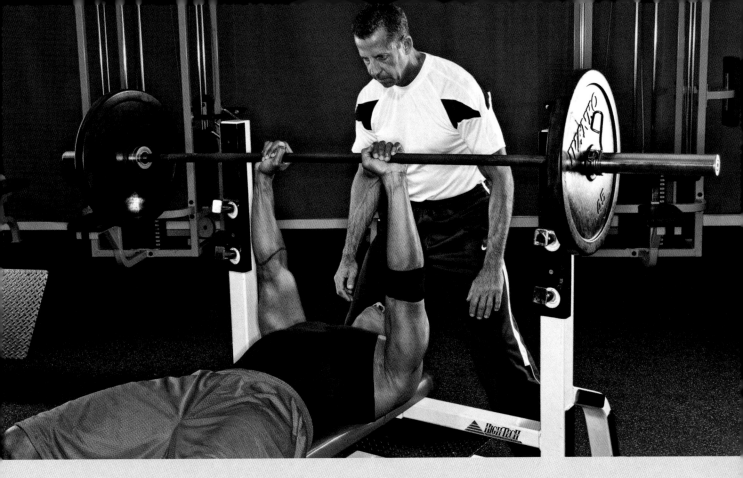

Close-Grip Bench Press: Lie back on a flat bench with your feet flat on the floor. Grasp the barbell with a narrow (inside shoulder-width) overhand grip. Press the bar up slightly to unrack it, and hold it above your chest with your arms extended. Lower the bar to your lower chest, keeping your elbows close to your body. When the bar approaches an inch or so away from your chest, pause and press the bar back up to the starting position.

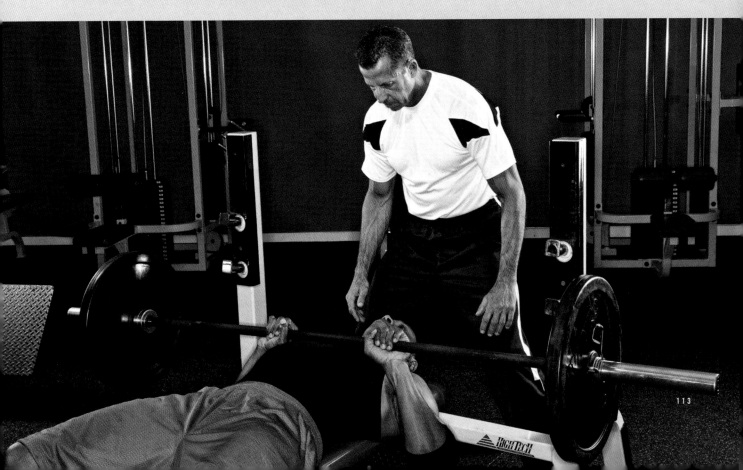

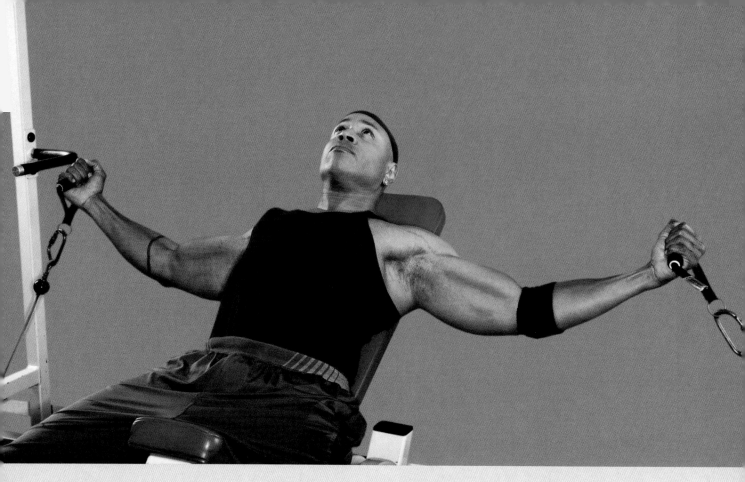

Incline-Bench Cable Fly: Place an incline bench equidistant between two low pulley cables. Grasp the two D-handles attached to the cables and lie flat on the bench. Keeping your arms slightly bent, pull the handles in front of you as if you were hugging a barrel, squeezing your chest when your hands are above your torso, then lower the handles to the start position, stopping when your upper arms are parallel to the bench.

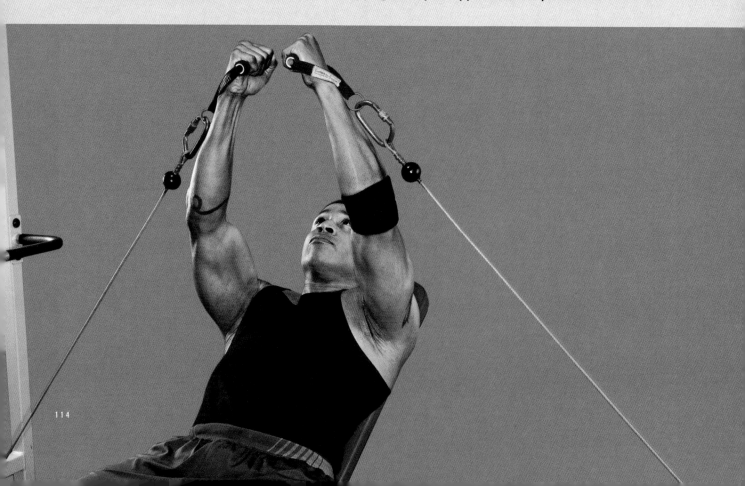

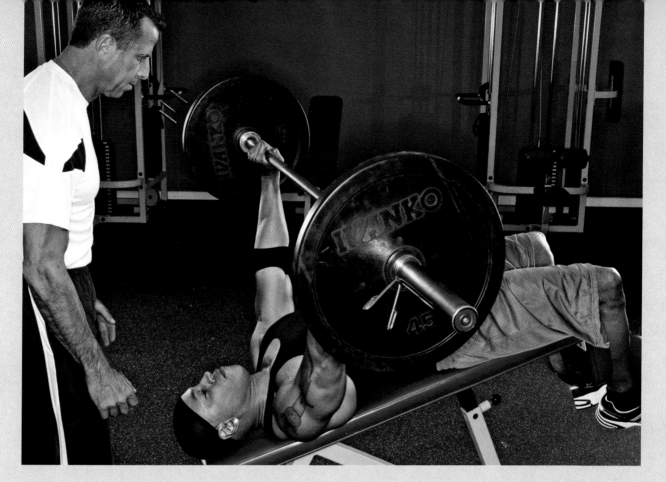

Decline Press: Lie faceup on a decline bench set at about a 45-degree angle. Your torso should be fully supported from your head to your hips, with your knees bent and feet supported. Grasp the bar with a wide, overhand grip. Bend your arms and slowly lower the bar toward your lower chest. When the bar reaches chest level, forcefully extend your arms, pressing the bar back to the start position.

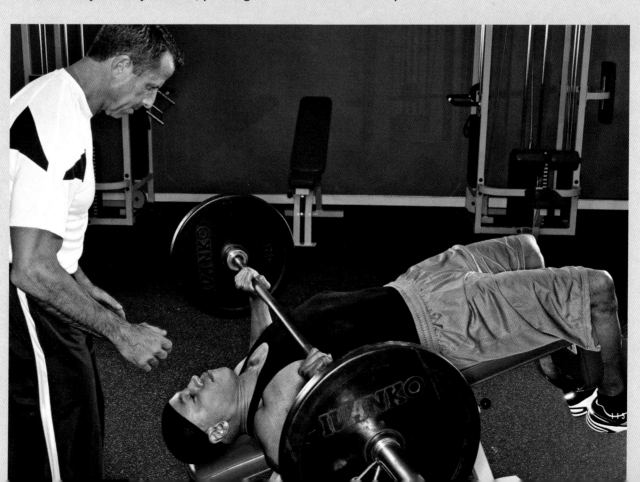

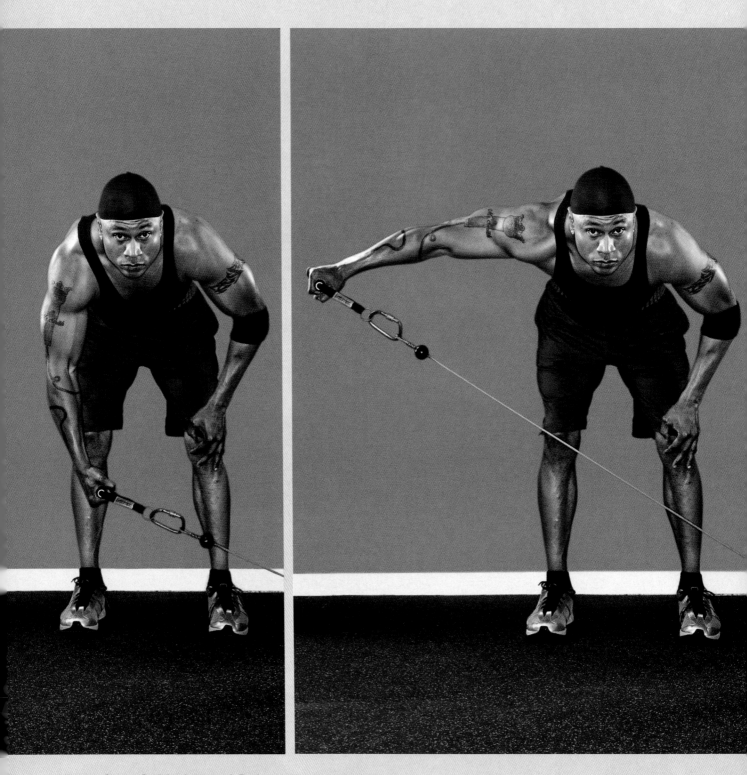

Bent-Over Cable Lateral Raise: With a D-handle in one hand, stand sideways to a low cable pulley, placing your nonworking hand on your knee or hip for balance. With your chest up, back flat, and knees slightly bent, bend over at the waist until your torso is just about parallel to the floor. Let the working arm hang directly beneath you with your elbow slightly bent. Keeping your arm bent, powerfully raise the cable up and out to your side until your upper arm is about parallel to your torso. Squeeze, then slowly lower your arm back to the start position.

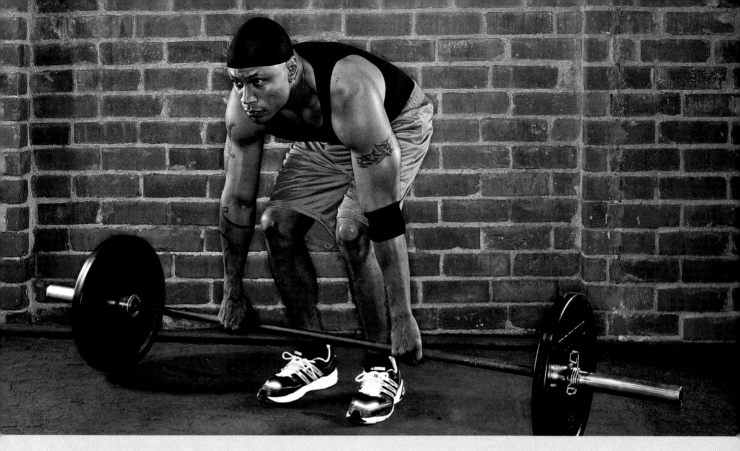

Deadlift: With your feet flat on the floor, squat down and grasp the bar with a slightly wider than shoulder-width grip. Allow the bar to rest flush against your shins. With your chest up and back flat, lift the bar by extending your hips and knees to full extension. Be sure to keep your arms straight throughout as you drag the bar up your legs until you reach a standing position. Squeeze your back, legs, and glutes, then lower the bar along the same path until it touches the floor. Allow the bar to settle for a second before beginning the next rep.

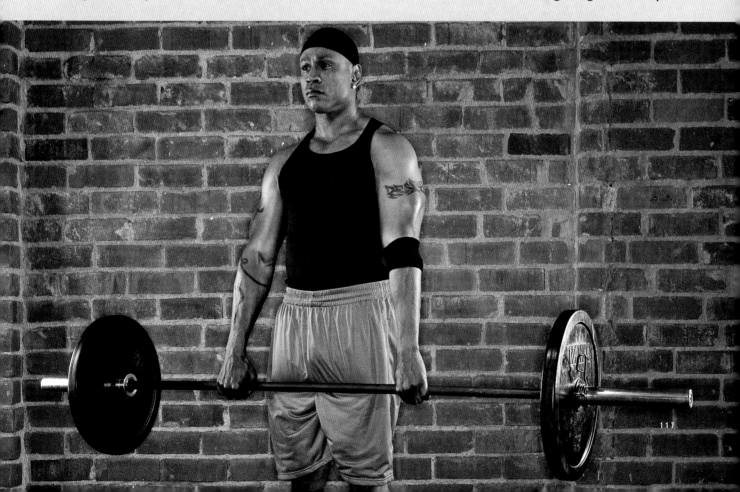

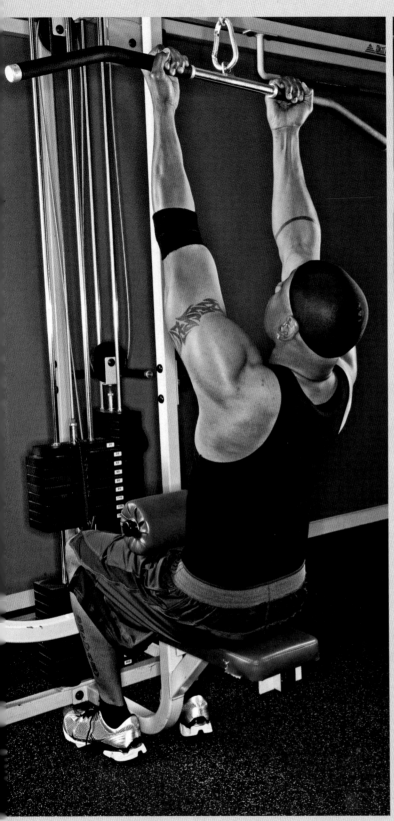
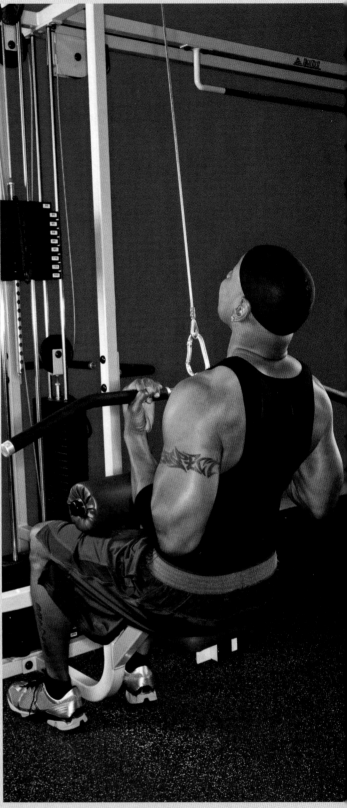

Reverse-Grip Lat Pulldown: Attach a long lat bar to the pulley and adjust the kneepad so that you fit snugly in the seat. Grasp the bar with a reverse, shoulder-width grip and sit down, maintaining an erect posture by contracting your lower back. Your arms should be fully extended above you with your head straight and feet flat on the floor. Contract your lats to pull the bar down to your upper chest, bringing your elbows as far behind you as possible. Squeeze your shoulder blades together at the bottom and slowly return the bar along the same path.

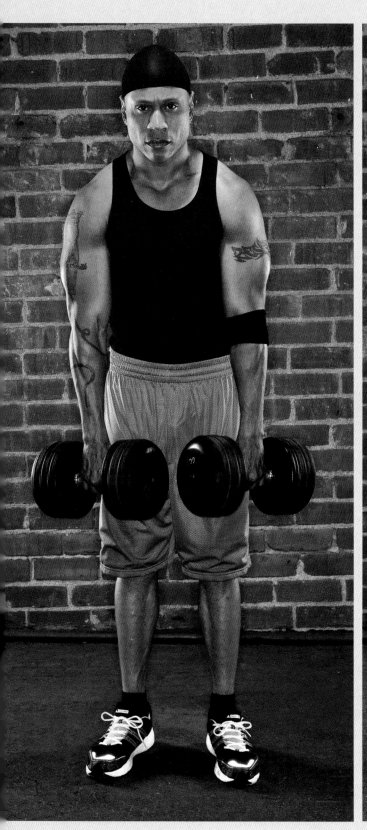 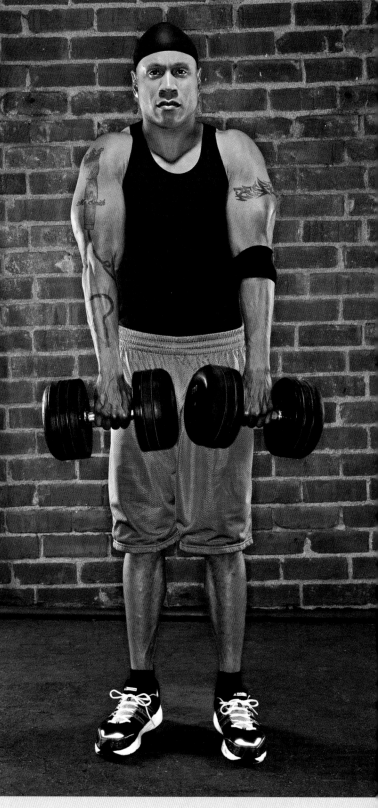

Dumbbell Shrug: Stand holding a dumbbell in each hand at your sides. Keeping your chest up and abs tight, shrug your shoulders straight up toward the ceiling, squeezing your traps at the top. Slowly reverse the motion to lower back to the start position.

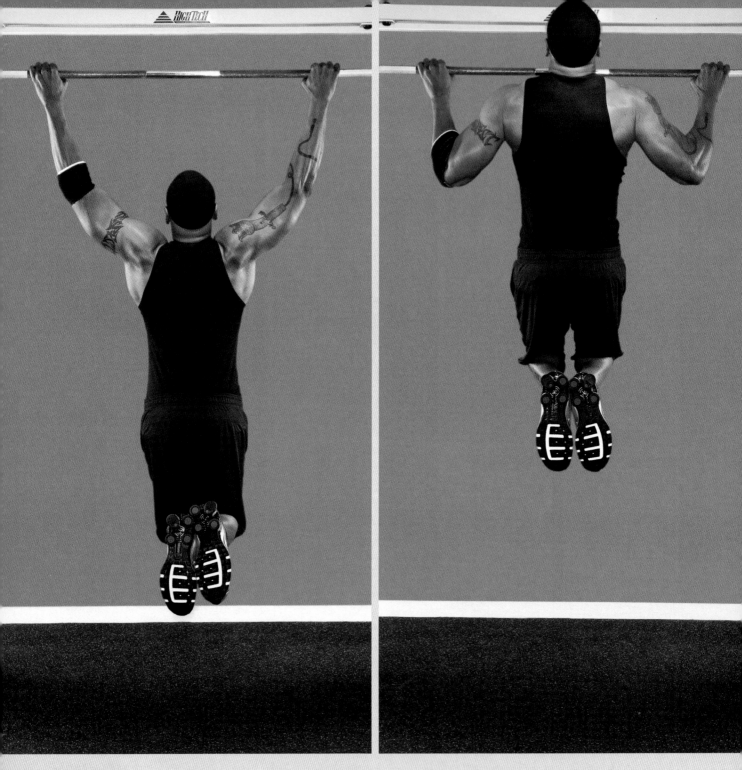

Pullup: Grasp a fixed overhead bar with a wide, overhand grip, your thumbs wrapped around the bar for safety. Hang freely from the bar, elbows fully extended and feet crossed behind you. Contract your lats to raise your chin over the bar, concentrating on keeping your elbows out to your sides and pulling them down to your sides to raise yourself. Hold momentarily in the peak contracted position before lowering yourself to the start position.

Machine Crunch (not pictured): Sit inside an ab machine with your arms across the pad. With your feet flat on the floor, flex your abs to crunch forward, moving the pad toward your knees. Squeeze and hold, then return to the start position. Don't allow the weight plates to touch down between reps.

SCOOTER'S 30-MINUTE WORKOUTS

Being on the Platinum 360 Plan is a real commitment, and I'm not gonna lie, 10 minutes in the morning won't get you Platinum results; you have to put in the time to see real change. But we all have days when there just isn't time to get it all done. Rather than give the gym a pass altogether, swap in one of these streamlined routines. Or perhaps you're traveling and you only have time for arms and abs before you head to your meeting. We have you covered. You might even want to link together two or more of these workouts to construct your own week-long plan, and that's fine, too. All of these mini-routines work hand-in-hand with the 360 Plan.

The great thing about these workouts is that they don't sacrifice results simply because you're in and out of the gym in 30 minutes. To the contrary, by increasing the intensity through super-sets and strategic combinations, you'll make your goals and maintain the progress you've made with the 360 Plan. How does it work? These 30-minute workouts are chockful of compound moves that direct more oxygen to working muscles and cause more calories to be burned. Since you have no time to waste, there's no wasted effort. As long as you put in the effort, you'll have the body you want in no time.

Legs, Delts

Exercise	Sets	Reps
Smith Squat (page 51)	2	10–12
superset with		
Upright Row (page 60)	2	10–12
Leg Press (page 33)	2	10–12
superset with		
Dumbbell Front Raise (page 90)	2	10–12
Lying Leg Curl (page 35)	2	10–12
superset with		
Seated Overhead Dumbbell Press (page 61)	2	10–12
Barbell Lunge (page 53)	2	10–12
superset with		
Bent-Over Cable Lateral Raise (page 116)	2	10–12
Split-Jump Squat (page 110)	2	To failure
superset with		
Jump Squat (page 105)	2	To failure

Rest 30 seconds between sets; does not include warmup sets.

Back, Hamstrings

Exercise	Sets	Reps
Lat Pulldown (page 36)	4	10–12
Seated Cable Row (page 47)	4	15–20
Romanian Deadlift (page 81)	4	8–10
Lying Leg Curl (page 35)	4	12–15
Lat Pulldown (repeat)	4	15–20
Rest 30 seconds between sets; does not include warmup sets.		

Upper Body, Abs

Exercise	Sets	Reps
Reverse-Grip Lat Pulldown (page 118)	2	12
superset with		
Seated Overhead Dumbbell Press (page 61)	2	12
Incline Cable Fly (page 58)	2	12
superset with		
Straight-Arm Pulldown (page 68)	2	12
Seated Cable Row (page 47)	2	12
superset with		
Flat-Bench Dumbbell Fly (page 79)	2	12
Barbell Curl (page 49)	2	12
superset with		
Lying Triceps Extension (page 107)	2	12
Hanging Knee Raise (page 86)	2	To failure
Rest 30 seconds between sets; does not include warmup sets.		

Lower Body, Abs, Core

Exercise	Sets	Reps
Barbell Squat (page 67)	3	15
superset with		
Leg Extension (page 34)	3	15
Leg Curl	2	15
superset with		
Hack Squat (page 67)	2	15
Leg Press (page 33)	2	15
superset with		
Romanian Deadlift (page 81)	2	15
Dumbbell Stepup (page 52)	2	15 (each leg)
Barbell Lunge (page 53)	2	15 (steps each leg)
Plank (hold the position at the top of a pushup)	2	To failure

Rest 30 seconds between sets; does not include warmup sets.

Arms, Calves, Abs

Exercise	Sets	Reps
Barbell Curl (page 49)	3	6, 8, 12
Close-Grip Bench Press (page 80)	3	6, 8, 12
Preacher Curl (page 104)	3	8, 10, 15
Reverse-Grip Pressdown (page 64)	3	8, 10, 15
Incline Cable Curl (page 106)	3	12, 15, 20
Overhead Cable Extension (page 66)	3	To failure
Standing Calf Raise (page 42)	2	30
Cable Crunch (page 50)	1	To failure

Rest 30 seconds between sets; does not include warmup sets.

Scooter's Tip

Take your recovery time as seriously as you do your training. When at rest, your muscles patch themselves and grow. If you constantly break them down without giving them a chance to rebuild, you'll never allow your body to respond and transform itself.

SCOOTER'S 30-MINUTE WORKOUT CHEAT SHEET

Full descriptions of these exercises appear elsewhere in this book. Please refer back if you need a reminder of how to perform any of them.

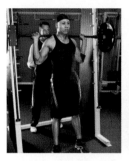 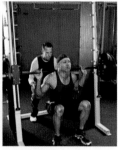

Smith Squat (p. 51)

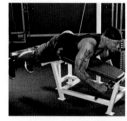 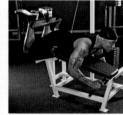

Lying Leg Curl (p. 35)

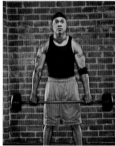 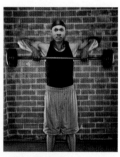

Upright Row (p. 60)

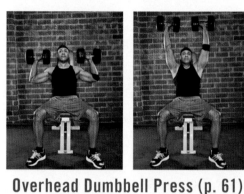 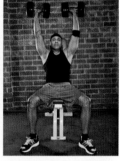

Overhead Dumbbell Press (p. 61)

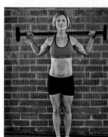 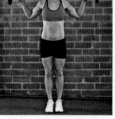 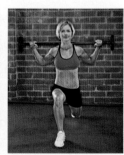

Leg Press (p. 33)

Barbell Lunge (p. 53)

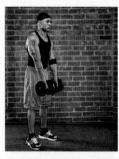 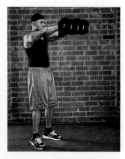

Dumbbell Front Raise (p. 90)

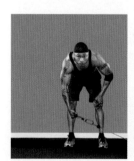 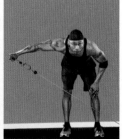

Bent-Over Cable Lateral Raise (p. 116)

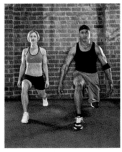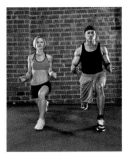

Split-Jump Squat (p. 110)

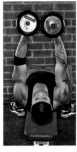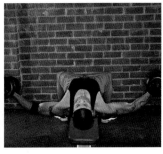

Flat-Bench Dumbbell Fly (p. 79)

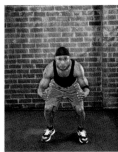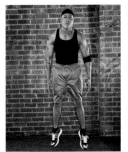

Jump Squat (p. 105)

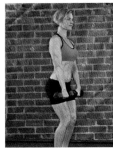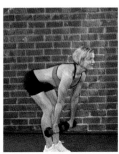

Romanian Deadlift (p. 81)

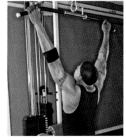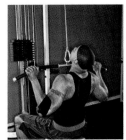

Lat Pulldown (p. 36)

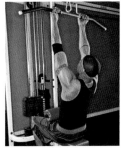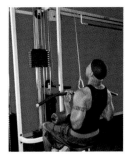

Reverse-Grip Lat Pulldown (p. 118)

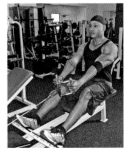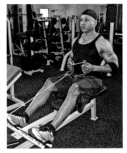

Seated Cable Row (p. 47)

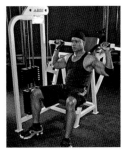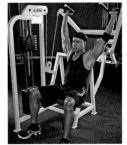

Overhead Machine Press (p. 39)

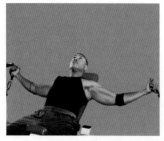
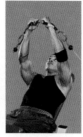

Incline Cable Fly (p. 58)

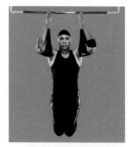
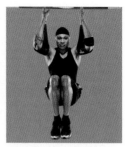

Hanging Knee Raise (p. 86)

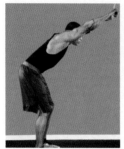
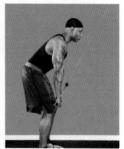

Straight-Arm Pulldown (p. 68)

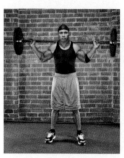
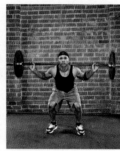

Barbell Squat (p. 67)

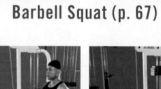

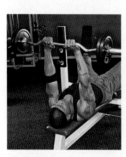
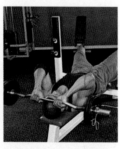

Barbell Curl (p. 49)

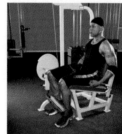
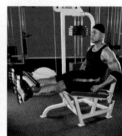

Leg Extension (p. 34)

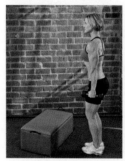
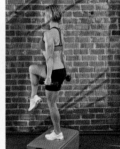

Lying Triceps Extension (p. 107)

Dumbbell Stepup (p. 52)

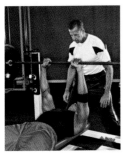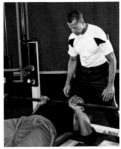

Close-Grip Bench Press (p. 80)

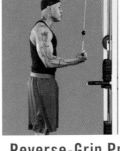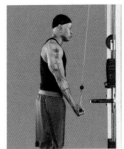

Reverse-Grip Pressdown (p. 64)

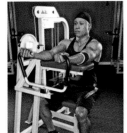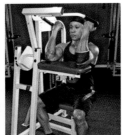

Preacher Curl (p. 104)

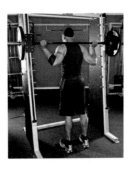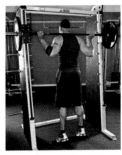

Standing Calf Raise (p. 42)

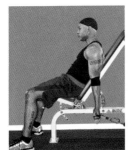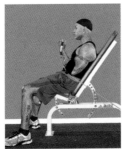

Incline Cable Curl (p. 106)

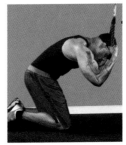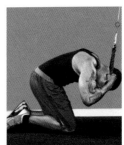

Cable Crunch (p. 50)

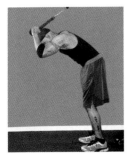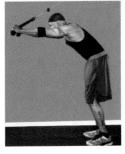

Overhead Cable Extension (p. 66)

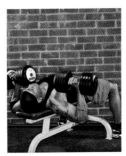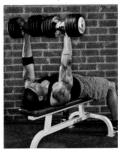

Dumbbell Bench Press (p. 57)

Hack Squat (p. 67)

PART THREE

THE
PLATINUM 360
NUTRITION PLAN

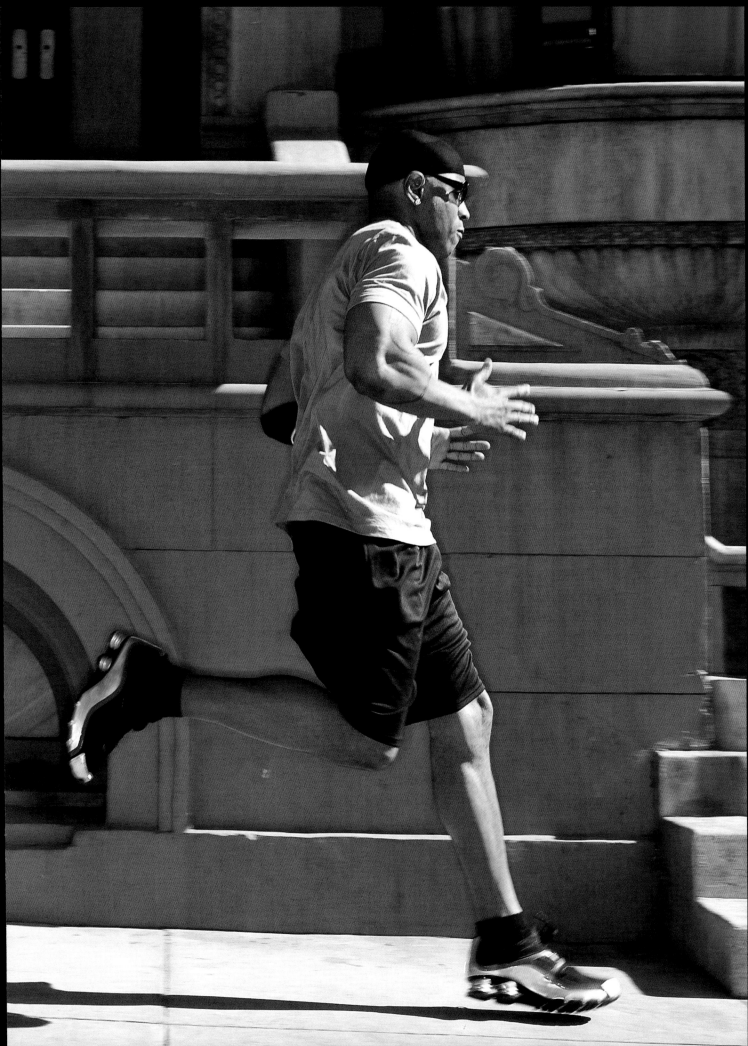

THE RIGHT FUEL FOR YOUR 360 TRANSFORMATION

You still here? Of course you are! Because our journey isn't complete; you have yet to come full circle. I know your muscles are sore and you have a lot on your mind from Parts One and Two, but that is all part of my plan for you. I set out to exercise and stimulate you from head to toe to get your mind and body on the same page. So let's pause for a minute to look back at what we've accomplished so far. When we started, we focused on creating the type of mind-set that would allow you to be a successful, open-minded, well-rounded person. Remember, the way I've designed my 360 plan isn't linear. If the first thing you want to do is get in the gym, pick up the book and flip to my Platinum 360 Workout. You can also go back to the first few chapters for reinforcement anytime. The ideas and lessons are timeless and can be applied at any phase of your journey: beginning, middle, or end. Actually, there is no true end; this is a life journey. Never stop improving. Never stop growing. Never stop getting better. If you are not getting better, you are getting worse.

You've been working on your body, now you need the right kind of fuel. Welcome to my Platinum 360 Nutrition Plan, which works hand in hand with the Platinum 360 Workout. Think of it less as a diet and more as a nutritional lifestyle. A diet is just something you try for a little while. If you've gotten this far, you're in it for more than just a little while.

So are you hungry? You gotta be. The Platinum 360 Workout is no joke. Put those keys down, though. We're not jumping in the car and heading off to the nearest fast-food joint for your favorite 1,200-calorie triple-stacked burger. That was the old you. The mirror only cares about the new you, and you haven't come full circle just yet. Learning what best fuels your lifestyle and sticking to the foods that are good for you while avoiding what's strictly off-limits requires patience and discipline, just like the Platinum Workout. I've said it once but I'll say it again: Nothing comes easy. You will feel the pain and you will suffer the burn. But pain on the way to a goal is a lot better than the pain that comes from failing to reach that goal. Right now your goal is achieving the body you desire and the improved health and fitness that come with it. I'm here to tell you that all is well within reach. Heck, you should already be feeling some changes by now. But working out is only half the equation. What you put into your body is the other half.

You have probably tried one diet or another—who hasn't? Maybe you've toyed with high-protein this and low-calorie that and failed to get the kind of results you were looking for. Good news: Here's where your fruitless search for the perfect nutrition plan ends. You've already seen what the workout can do for you. Wait until you see the result you get when you combine that with a diet regimen specifically designed to complement the workout, giving you just the right combination of protein, carbs, and energy to give you the optimal benefits. Believe me, I know from my own experience, the results speak for themselves. But enough about me; this is all about you.

Knowledge is power. What do you really know about food? Part of the reason other diets have failed you is because you didn't fully understand the science behind them and how certain foods work with your body chemistry to keep your metabolism running efficiently. Without this knowledge, it's hard to make good food choices. My nutrition plan explains exactly how carbs, protein,

fats, and other nutritional components really work in your body. Armed with that understanding, you're much more likely to eat intelligently and ultimately get more out of the plan.

I love to eat, as many people who have seen me in fancy restaurants will attest. I know you do, too. But eating whatever, you want and hoping for that perfect body is an exercise in futility. Even if you follow the Platinum Workout plan to a T, you won't achieve optimal results if you eat an ice-cream sundae every night. This book is about maximizing every last bit of your potential, and you can't do that on a diet of empty calories and processed foods. But don't worry, eating right doesn't mean depriving yourself indefinitely of the things you love. Discipline, moderation, and knowledge of what you eat and how food works are the keys to implementing the Platinum 360 Nutrition Plan successfully.

From this point forward, you will be smarter about how you eat. Being smarter means being healthier. And yeah, what you start to see in the mirror will make it all worthwhile. Take one last look at those extra pounds you've been trying to shed. Say good-bye.

CHAPTER 6
WHY THE PLATINUM 360 NUTRITION PLAN WORKS

The Platinum 360 Nutrition Plan is the perfect complement to the Platinum 360 Workout Plan, and each of its phases is designed to work in tandem with the corresponding phase of the workout, so that as you get stronger, you get leaner and healthier, too. The best part is that this nutrition plan isn't about what you shouldn't do, it's about what you *should* do.

Everybody loves to eat. Let's face it, eating is a great part of the human experience. Don't get me started about Thai food. Or Japanese. Or Italian. Or Mom's cooking. But food is more than just a way to satisfy hunger and bring people together. What you put in your system helps you create your life. It feeds your mind and your soul, as well as your body. When you're on my nutrition plan, you'll have more brainpower; you'll have more energy when you go to the gym; you'll have more spark for the rest of your day;

you'll realize you're in a better mood. In short, you will function and feel better. And all this while getting your eat on.

I've heard people say they wish there was a magic pill to help them get to the body weight they want overnight. If there were? Hey, sign me up! It would save a whole lot of time, wouldn't it? But since we both know there is no magic pill, the best choice we can make is to embrace the process and the journey. Working out and eating right are lifestyle choices that make us who we are. You want magic? The closest thing to real magic is the book you are holding in your hand . . .

Parts 2 and 3 of the Platinum program—training and nutrition—work hand-in-hand. If you work out without following a proper nutrition plan, you won't get the results you're looking for. If you cut your calories but don't work out, you may lose weight, but you'll probably just end up burning muscle instead of fat. Ultimately, you aren't going to be as happy with the way you look or the way you feel if you don't hit some iron and get your butt moving while you're eating right. This isn't a get-fit-quick scheme. This is about devoting yourself to getting it right and keeping it tight.

LEARNING THE BASICS

Before I give you the rundown on what you need to do to follow my 8-week nutrition plan, let me get in Cornel West mode and school you on the building blocks of nutrition. You gotta know a little about food and its effects on your body—metabolism, anyone?—so that you'll know why the program is actually working.

Peep this: You go on a diet, cut back on what you eat, and maintain that discipline for a couple of weeks. You go to bed hungry; you haul your butt up out of bed to get to the gym before you go to work; you sweat, you get sore, and now you're starting to feel pretty good about yourself. Maybe you even drop a few pounds. All of a sudden, the jeans in the back of your closet fit like a glove. You look in the mirror and say, "I'm the bomb!" But after a couple of weeks, you realize it's too much. The morning comes and your alarm blasts your ears like a drum. You hit the snooze button and it's back to dreamland. Finally, you get up late, grab a couple of donuts like you're Homer Simpson, and feel terrible for the rest of the day. The next day you have less energy than the day before. Pretty soon, you're right back where you started—if you're lucky. Many people rebound to the point where they look and feel even worse than they did before they started their ridiculous super-low-calorie diets.

So, what's up?

The problem is those diets are cheating you like a card shark on a street corner. *When you push too hard physically and emotionally while depriving your body of its basic needs, you're going down for sure.*

You need to get real. You probably know that protein, carbs, and fats are the basic components of food. You probably also know that protein supports muscle building and that carbs and fats provide energy. But here's something you may not know. There are some big differences within these groups. Different forms of protein and fats can have minor effects on how your body looks and feels, but the biggest difference in your diet has to do with how many and what type of carbs you give to your body at specific times of the day and week.

All the foods you eat provide your body with energy in the form of calories. Because fats have more calories per gram than protein or carbs do, they sometimes get a bad rap. However, all three can play an important role in helping you boost your energy levels while cutting back on your stored body fat *if* you know how much of each to eat and when.

Here we go. Class is in session.

Calories— Boosting Your Metabolism

When you get right down to it, adding and losing weight is some pretty simple old-school math: calories in versus calories out. But it can be tricky trying to get your body to zap fat, and you need excess body fat like you need a kick in the head. If you jump on a treadmill and run like you're Forrest Gump, there's a good chance that you'll be burning muscle instead of fat. Not cool, people. What's the solution? You need to *train* your body to burn body fat. One way you do that is through a proper balance of cardio and weight training. The other way is by giving your body the nutrients it needs for each phase of your day, and each kind of workout, to keep it performing at its fat-burning peak.

The sweetest thing about my nutrition plan is that it cranks up your metabolic rate—which means you'll be nuking fat all day long. For real! The more calories you burn, the more weight you're going to lose. So, there are two ways to ramp up the number of calories your body burns each day: (1) get active (that little army of fat cells loves when you sit on the couch), and (2) boost your metabolic rate so

that your body burns more calories while you're resting. Since there are only so many hours in a day, and girl, I know you're busy, it's tough to get much time in the gym. So stepping up the amount of calories you burn while doing your normal daily activities is mad important. Without it, long-term success is only a dream.

Here are some of the best ways to say goodbye to that fat without damaging precious muscle.

- **Don't neglect weight training.**

  Most people think that putting in extra hours on the elliptical machine or treadmill is the fastest route to weight loss, but while cardio does help burn fat, that's only part of the story. There's nothing like hitting iron, because your muscles continue to use energy to recover from a weight workout. That's why you end up burning extra calories for up to *2 days* after a weight workout. Can y'all say bonus? The more muscle mass you have, the more calories your body burns, even while you're chilling in your recliner or reading that guilty-pleasure novel poolside. You should work out with weights at least three times a week. Follow the weight training plans in Part Two, and you'll keep your metabolic rate sky high by *maintaining or even adding muscle mass.*

- **Perform aerobic activity.**

  Like I said, if you get on a treadmill and just go, you may burn muscle mass along with body fat. But trust me, cardio is still your friend. You definitely want to include aerobic activity in your training plan. Aerobic exercise is a beast because it uses a large portion of the body's muscle mass, such as the legs, back, and even arms. When you include cardio in your workout after your weight training, you fire up both calorie- and body fat–burning. Don't get mad if you're turning heads in no time.

- **Eat plenty of protein at every meal.**

What do you know about the thermic effect of food? Sounds crazy, huh? But it's the number of calories your body burns after consuming food. But some foods really ratchet up this effect more than others. That bod of yours uses more calories to digest protein than it does carbs or fats. Protein ain't no joke—it contains a little less than 4 calories per gram—so it takes your body more calories to process it. So if a diet is high in lean protein, it'll pump up that metabolic rate. You don't need to explain that to anybody; they'll know it when they see how good you look.

- **Avoid eating large amounts of carbs, especially processed carbs.**

Here's the deal: Protein has a thermic effect. But carbs? Not so much. The worst offenders are processed carbs, especially sugar and white flour. When you eat a lot of these foods without much protein and fats to balance them, your body releases a lot of insulin. You don't want that. Insulin takes carbs and quickly converts them to fat. It also slows down fat burning, so it's jacking you two times. If you're throwing down on a huge baked potato or big bowl of pasta, you're providing your body with way more carb energy than it needs for the next couple hours. You know how you feel like you want to go to sleep after killing

some pasta? That's the insulin talking. And it's not asking you to hit the club. It's saying, "Hey, time for you to pack on the pounds."

- **Spice up your meals.**

One of the best ways to boost your metabolism is to add spices to your meals. Throw in some zest to keep it interesting. Add crushed red pepper to chicken breasts or fish before cooking; add hot sauce to your eggs or spicy salsa to cottage cheese. All these bad boys are well worth the negligible calories they add to your eats.

- **Eat fatty fish.**

Fish such as salmon, trout, tuna, and arctic char are rich in essential omega-3 fats. Good thing. These fats tend to increase fat burning. Try to eat fatty fish two to three times per week. It's not only tasty, but it will bust up fat that's stored in your body.

- **Drink green tea.**

The active ingredient in green tea, epigallocatechin gallate (EGCG), helps jack up your metabolism. Step it up a notch by adding lemon juice to your green tea to boost the amount of EGCG your body absorbs. That'll make the tea even more effective. See how simple that was?

- **Stay hydrated.**

You know you gotta drink up. But you may not know that drinking plenty of water also helps you burn more fat when you're working out. Drinking two 8-ounce glasses of cold water can boost metabolic rate by about 30 percent. Weight loss doesn't get much easier than that. Drink 16 ounces of cold water between meals and before, during, and after working out. So bottoms up.

Protein—Feed Your Muscles and Your Body

If it's not already, protein should be your new best friend. Protein is an integral part of your nutrition plan. It builds muscles, gives you energy, and pumps up your metabolic rate. In short, it's a beast. Just like fats and carbs, protein can be used as immediate energy when amino acids, the small building-block molecules that are crucial for growth and that make up protein, are converted into carbohydrate energy. It takes your body longer to break protein down into fuel that your body can use immediately, but it can be super-useful.

Check these protein tips.

- **Get enough protein every day.**

  You need lots of protein throughout the day, every day, all day. Whether you're a 120-pound woman or a 200-pound man, you need at least a gram of protein for every pound of body weight. That's about 25 grams of protein per meal on average for a person under 150 pounds, about 30 grams of protein for someone between 150 to 200 pounds, and 35 grams of protein for someone over 200 pounds. You can take in more, of course, but beyond a certain point (more than 35 grams per meal), excess protein will be converted to energy instead of being used for repair and recovery. Translation: Get enough, but don't overdo it. Shoot for a gram per pound of your body weight, and you'll be good to go.

- **Include protein in every meal.**

  You want to make sure your body gets a steady flow of protein throughout the day. Since protein takes a few hours to digest fully, a good dose every 2 to 3 hours guarantees a continual supply of amino acids is delivered to your bloodstream. Don't get into the habit of going long stretches without feeding your body—and your muscles—another dose of protein. If you don't, your body will start breaking down your muscle mass for stored aminos. And you'll be waving bye-bye to that lean muscle you are working so hard to build.

- **Eat protein before you go to bed.**

  Load up before you hit the pillow. You fast while you sleep, so your body has to get fuel from somewhere. Muscle is an easy target. Taking in a small amount of protein with some fats or fiber before you go to bed helps to provide a slow, steady release of amino acids while you're off in dreamland. Your muscles can't protect themselves at night. It's up to you to get their back with a quick hit of protein before you call it a night.

- **Take in protein before and after you work out.**

  Your body's need for amino acids shoots up when you hit the weights. By eating a meal that's high in protein no more than an hour before you start your workout, you're ensuring that you have the necessary nutrients for energy during the workout and for building and repairing your body after stressing it. This goes back to our tip about getting a steady stream of protein so you're constantly feeding your muscles.

- **Emphasize a spectrum of protein foods.**

  You wouldn't wear the same thing every day, would you? No, you mix and match and coordinate. Now do the same thing with your protein. You often hear people argue about what form of protein is "best"—eggs, soy, dairy, lean meats, or fish. I'm here to tell you that you're much better off mixing it up from meal to meal, from day to day, because some proteins are high in certain amino acids and low in others. By mixing and matching your proteins, you'll get sufficient amounts of each. Getting multiple protein sources will ensure you're getting a good blend of amino acids. Get creative, people.

Carbs—Provide Fuel in Fast- and Slow-Digesting Forms

All this talk about protein may make it seem like you should avoid carbs altogether. That would make for a pretty simple diet plan— just eat meat and other sources of pure protein, with a little fat thrown in for good measure. But you need carbs, too. Carbs are your friend as long as you take in the right kind.

Foods that are high in carbs essentially fall into one of two categories: fast-digesting and slow-digesting (kind of like East Coast and West Coast rappers). Sugar and most starchy carbs are fast-digesting. When you pop that orange drink from the corner store or polish off a bagel (with your favorite jelly) from the deli up the street, your body will digest it quickly, and you'll experience a rapid rise in blood sugar levels and a big insulin spike. This will lock down your fat burning like a flypaper defender. Boom. Fat 1, you 0. This is especially true when you eat carbs without any protein, fats, or fiber, all of which slow down the digestive process.

The good news is that many carbs are slow-digesting. These include high-fiber foods like vegetables, many fruits, and whole grain foods like oatmeal, brown rice, and whole grain breads. Because these carbs digest slowly, they do not result in quick spikes in blood sugar and insulin and therefore help to burn fat all day long.

All carbs, whether they are slow- or fast-digesting, are holding down about 4 calories per gram. But with the slow-digesting type, fewer carbs reach your bloodstream over the course of the day, almost like they're stuck on the Long Island Expressway. Oftentimes, athletes who consume slow-digesting carbs have more energy throughout the day. Come on. Who couldn't use more energy? So it's a win-win situation with slow carbs—you burn more body fat *and* have more energy. Take that, fat. Bam!

Let's jump into the basics.

- **Get in some slow-digesting carbs when you wake up.**

    When you crawl out of bed in the morning, your blood sugar is way down. So after you hit the shower, sit down at the breakfast table and make sure you have some slow-digesting carbs in front of you. Good choices include fruit, oatmeal, and whole grain products such as bagels, bread, or pancakes. I'm guessing those have been on your menu for a while. These slow-digesting carbs will hook you up with a steady release of energy that won't spike your insulin too high. They won't help you catch that bus to work, though. You're on your own with that one.

- **Eat fruits and vegetables throughout the day.**

   Turns out Moms was right after all. Fruits and veggies are the joint. They are low in calories, loaded with nutrients, and they digest slowly. Eat them with every meal. Don't worry about the carbs they have—the carbs in vegetables and fruits have little impact on insulin release. So you're good.

   Another plus: Fruits and vegetables contain mad fiber, so they digest slowly. Aim for no more than 2 to 3 pieces of fruit a day and at least 5 or 6 servings of vegetables. And, hey, you might even meet that special someone in the produce section. Wink.

- **Take in fast-digesting carbs after workouts.**

   What? Not carbs again. I know you're thinking I told you to stay away from them. But fast-digesting carbs do serve a purpose. In addition to being readily stored as body fat, they are also stored as muscle glycogen, a fancy word for the carbohydrates that are stored in your muscles.

   When you work out, you burn the carbs that are stored in your muscles as glycogen. You need to restore that as soon as possible to (1) provide your muscles with the nutrients they need for recovery and growth, and (2) make sure the next time you work out, your muscles will have proper levels of glycogen. Now pay attention here: Immediately after your workout is the one time your body will not use fast-digesting carbs against you. So, if you crave foods with sugar, now is the time to cheat. This get-out-of-jail-free card is only

good for 30 minutes after your workouts, though. Act fast, and try not to get crumbs everywhere.

- **Get plenty of fiber.**

   If you know anything about healthy eating (at this point in the book you know a ton), then you probably know that fiber is very important. Like, seatbelt important. Although fiber is made up of carbohydrates, it's a nondigestible form of carbs, so it does not increase insulin release because it can't be absorbed through the lining of your digestive tract. So although you've consumed the fiber, it doesn't truly "enter" your body (another dinner party jewel).

   Fiber can be pretty helpful. It cleans your digestive system, helps slow the absorption (and thus the insulin release) of other foods, and also carries some foods through your body, preventing them from being absorbed. Didn't realize fiber was that busy, huh?

   Because nutritional labeling on packaged food includes fiber in the total carb count—even though it is never absorbed—you can subtract the amount of fiber from the total amount of carbs. For example, a high-fiber carb source that contains 20 grams of total carbs, 5 grams of which are fiber, actually provides you with only 15 grams of carbs. Now there's some math we can all agree with.

- **Avoid carbs before bedtime.**

   Most people are far less active in the evening than during the daytime. And since your insulin sensitivity tends to decrease in the evening, the carbs you get later in the day are less likely to be burned for energy and more likely to be stored as body fat. Bad news if you're trying to fit into that new bathing suit, girl. So your last two meals of the day—dinner and late-night snack—should be low in carbs. Sure, it goes without saying, but I know you like the sound of my voice in your head.

Fats—Give Your Body, Mind, and Soul What They Need to Feel Complete

Dietary fats get a bad rap, but that's not entirely fair. Many fad diets of the past eliminated too much dietary fat. The thinking was that if you cut out dietary fat, which contains more calories per ounce than protein or carbs, you'd cut down body fat. Makes sense, right? But many people overate low-fat carbs, causing their bodies to store fat like crazy.

Eating dietary fats in moderation doesn't translate to adding body fat, and in the proper amounts, some fats can even help you avoid adding body fat. Peace out, love handles. Even though fats are caloric, containing 9 calories for every gram (compared with about 4 calories per gram for protein), you can get a lot of bang for your buck. Dietary fats take a long time to digest, so when you take in a moderate amount, they help keep you from getting hungry, especially when compared with fast-digesting carbs.

Since dietary fats constantly get a bum rap, here's the real deal.

- **At least half your fats should come from unsaturated sources.**

    Some unsaturated fats are super-healthy.

Good examples are the fats found in avocados, nuts, seeds, olive and canola oils, and polyunsaturated omega-3 fats, such as those in fatty fish like salmon, trout, tuna, and arctic char. Gotta give a shoutout to flaxseed and walnuts, too.

Monounsaturated fats can help to lower cholesterol and, therefore, your risk of heart disease. If it protects that ticker of yours, that's good news. Peep this: These fats are readily used during exercise and not stored as body fat. Folks who increase their monounsaturated fat intake lose weight without actually reducing their calorie intake. Omega-3 fats are essential because your body cannot make them on its own. These fats not only increase fat burning but also can enhance joint and muscle recovery, prevent depression, and reduce the risk of heart disease and certain cancers. Talk about multitasking. Bet you didn't know fat had that type of game.

- **Don't fear saturated fats.**

    If unsaturated fats are good for you, then saturated fats must be bad, right? These fats are often solid at room temperature and are found in such foods as eggs, dairy, and meat. When you take in too much saturated fat, these large fat molecules can float around in your body for too long, driving up cholesterol levels and creating risk factors for heart disease and other problems you don't want any part of. Simple solution: Avoid chowing down on tons of saturated fats.

    But get this: These saturated fats play critical roles at all times. You need saturated fats to help keep you from feeling depleted and weak. They're big time when it comes to the building blocks for important body chemicals such as hormones. Fact: Without saturated fats, a man's testosterone levels will decline, as will his muscle mass. And that ain't what we're shooting for.

- **Avoid trans fats.**

    Fats aren't all good. So, which fats *should* you avoid? The ones chemically altered to imitate saturated fats (i.e., solid at room temperature). These are often listed on food labels as hydrogenated oil or partially hydrogenated oil. No good, my friends. Trans fats have been implicated in heart disease, diabetes, certain cancers, and even Alzheimer's disease. We're trying to get healthy here, not drive up healthcare costs. The good news is that it is getting easier and easier to avoid these harmful fats, as they are becoming increasingly eliminated from many products. To steer clear of trans fats, avoid fried foods and packaged bakery goods. You know that drive-thru on the corner? Keep driving.

- **Eat fats to increase absorption of antioxidants.**

    Fats help your body absorb antioxidants. When you eat a salad with fat-free dressing, you don't absorb as much of the beneficial antioxidants from the salad as you do when you eat it with a full-fat dressing or with avocado added. We're keeping it simple here. So when eating salads, go with olive oil–based dressings, or add avocados, nuts, or fatty fish to your salad.

- **Eat fats when you want to slow digestion.**

    Including a little bit of dietary fat in your breakfast, lunch, dinner, and between-meal snacks will make your calories go a little further, meaning that you won't get hungry before it's time to eat again. This is true for both saturated and unsaturated fats, so the best idea is to eat a balance of the two.

- **Avoid fats when you want to speed up digestion.**

    Sometimes you want to kick your digestion up to another gear, such as before and after your workouts. The goal is to deliver protein to your muscles as quickly as possible. Problem: While carbs speed this up, fats slow it down. Eating a high-fat meal before working out can reduce blood flow to your exercising muscles, giving them less oxygen and nutrients when they are needed the most. So kick those fats to the curb before and after you work out.

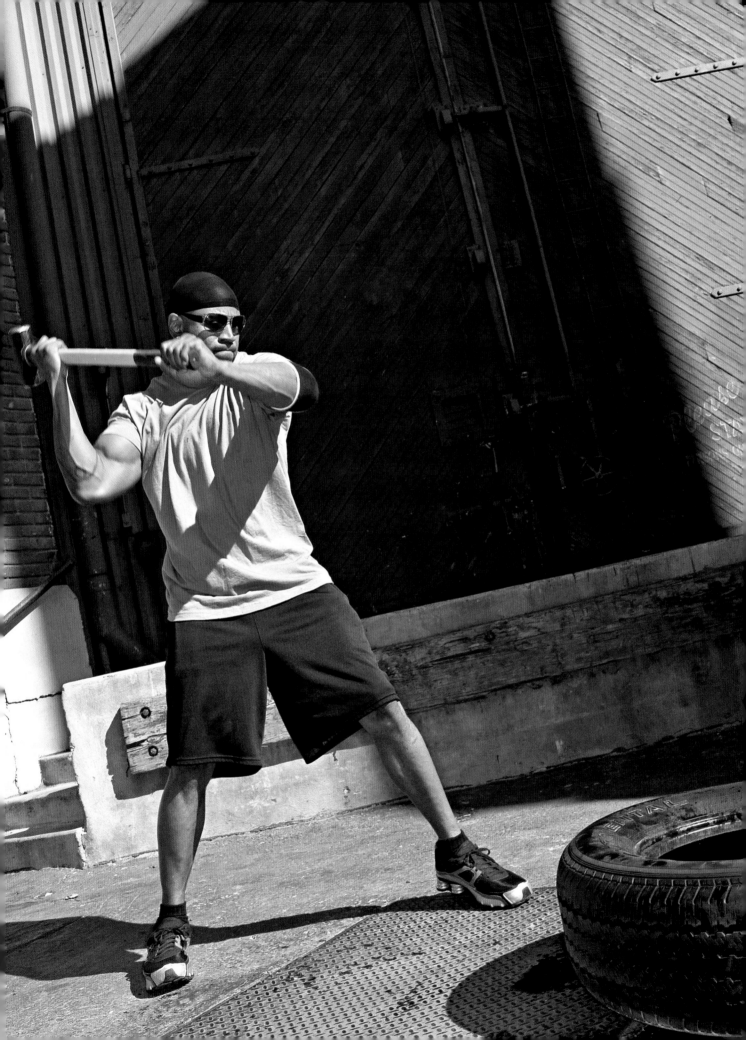

CHAPTER 7

THE PLATINUM 360 8-WEEK NUTRITION PLAN

Now you have a pretty good understanding of how your body responds to the foods that you eat and why it uses nutrients differently at different times of the day. So how do you use this information to design a program that maximizes your results at the gym? I thought you'd ask.

My nutrition program shifts macronutrients (you'll come to love that word) throughout the week—even over the course of a single day—so you can take advantage of the benefits each provides when it's needed the most, without taking in excess calories that will keep you from burning stored body fat. Best of all, at some point during any week, you will be able to eat just about any food you want. Try that on a "diet."

The plan is based on five different macronutrient strategies. These are:

- **Healthy Eating:** moderate carbs, moderate fats, high protein
- **Turbocharged Fat Burning:** low carbs, high fats, high protein
- **Calorie Restriction:** no carbs, low fats, high protein
- **Cheat Meal:** high carbs, high fats, high protein
- **Carb Refuel:** high carbs, low fats, high protein

Every meal on the 8-week plan that follows falls into one of these specific categories, so every meal that you eat is helping you work toward your health and fitness goal in a very strategic way. If you don't want to count calories and macronutrients, you don't have to. All you need to do is choose from the meal options for your weight level: under 150 pounds, 150 to 200 pounds, 200 pounds or more. Keep in mind that as you lose weight, you may need to drop down a level to make certain you're consuming the right amount of food for your ultimate goal.

On this meal plan, you can eat anything you want at some point during the week. Do you want chocolate? Crave an ice cold beer? Want some ice cream or a loaded pizza? Any of these can be part of your Saturday night Cheat Meal. If you like sugary carbs, you'll look forward to your Sunday Carb Refuel—a time of the week when you're encouraged to include fast-digesting carbs to help restock the glycogen stores that were depleted from your workouts and the low- and no-carb days earlier in the week.

If you don't want to choose from among the meal options or recipes I've provided on pages 176 to 218, but you still want to keep close tabs on everything you eat (a practice I highly recommend), start a food journal in which you record all the food that you eat, noting the amounts, the calories, and the macronutrient counts. This is an especially good idea when you are beginning the program and becoming comfortable with the idea of changing up the amounts of macros and calories you consume each day. To keep an accurate count of all this information, I recommend the following resources.

- Information taken from the ingredient panels on any packaged foods you eat (many national restaurant chains also provide nutritional information for their meals)
- The USDA Web site, which lists almost every food: http://www.nal.usda.gov/fnic/foodcomp/search/
- *The Complete Book of Food Counts* by Corinne T. Netzer

On the other hand, I know that's a lot of numbers, and you didn't sign up for math class. If you find it easier, just choose appropriate meals for your body weight from the meal options provided, or make appropriate substitutions based on the recipes.

THE MACRONUTRIENT STRATEGIES

This plan consists of four 2-week modules, followed by a maintenance plan you can stay on as long as you like. For the first 2 weeks, you'll follow the moderate-carb Healthy Eating program for 3 days, followed by 2 Turbocharged Fat Burning days with low carbs and higher fats. For most people, this will cover the weekdays of Monday through Friday, bringing you to your weekend strategy. For most of Saturday, you'll go no-carb Calorie Restriction—right up until your Cheat Meal at the end of the day. On Sunday, you cut the fat with a Carb Refuel day, which allows you to eat large quantities of carbs, even some of the processed types you shunned the rest of the week.

KEY TO THE PLATINUM 360 NUTRITION PLAN MACRONUTRIENT STRATEGIES

HEALTHY EATING: Moderate carbs, moderate fat, high protein

TURBOCHARGED FAT BURNING: Low carbs, high fat, high protein

CALORIE RESTRICTION: No carbs, low fat, high protein

CHEAT MEAL: High carbs, high fat, moderate protein

CARB REFUEL: High carbs, low fat, high protein

This Saturday and Sunday strategy is a constant throughout the 8-week plan. During Weeks 3 and 4, however, Day 3 switches from a Healthy Eating day to a Turbocharged Fat Burning day. This reduces your weekly carb consumption a bit, encouraging your body to keep burning body fat even as your metabolism revs up from the cardio and weight training, as well as the nutrients you're providing it from fats and protein and your weekend Carb Refuel. During Weeks 5 and 6, you add yet another Turbocharged Fat Burning day so that you are now following the Healthy Eating plan just 1 day a week and the Turbocharged Fat Burning for 4

days a week. By then, you will have reduced your overall intake of carbs substantially, forcing your body to rely more and more on body fat as an important fuel source. At this point in the program, your recovery Cheat Meal and Carb Refuel days play an even more crucial role in restocking your muscle glycogen stores and keeping your metabolic rate revved up through the long period of low to no carbs. Since your body will be even more depleted, this break from dieting will have a powerful effect on your metabolic rate, revving it up substantially.

Meals during Weeks 7 and 8 are very low in carbs. As you follow the Turbocharged Fat Burning plan from Monday to Friday, your Cheat Meal and Carb Refuel are crucial to keeping your metabolic rate elevated, so be certain that you take advantage of this time to eat the appropriate amount of carbs. They will not only taste great but also serve a crucial role in providing you with energy through the low- to no-carb phases that last from Monday morning through Saturday evening.

Once you've completed all 8 weeks of the plan, I hope you will go on the maintenance plan. It will help you continue to lose body fat while supplying the right amount of calories and nutrients to support your new body weight. After all, you don't want to pull the fatty weeds off your belly and have them grow right back. The maintenance plan will help you cut them off at the roots. If you haven't quite reached your target weight after 8 weeks on the Platinum 360 Nutrition Plan, you can repeat the entire 8-week plan after a 2-week break on the maintenance plan, then cycle through Weeks 3 through 8 again. Repeat this process as many times as it takes to get where you want to be, then stick with the maintenance program. Period. Smile.

THE PLATINUM 360 8-WEEK NUTRITION PLAN

Just like the Platinum 360 Workout, my nutrition plan changes as you progress. Here are the strategies you'll be following, broken down week by week. The meal choices that follow are designed to help you understand good options for each particular meal. Feel free to substitute your own favorites, or choose among the recipes in the next chapter. They are labeled by eating plan, so you can get more creative in the kitchen without blowing it in the dining room. And your scale will thank you.

Weeks 1 and 2

Monday	Healthy Eating
Tuesday	Healthy Eating
Wednesday	Healthy Eating
Thursday	Turbocharged Fat Burning
Friday	Turbocharged Fat Burning
Saturday	Calorie Restriction
Saturday night	Cheat Meal
Sunday	Carb Refuel

Weeks 3 and 4

Monday	Healthy Eating
Tuesday	Healthy Eating
Wednesday	Turbocharged Fat Burning
Thursday	Turbocharged Fat Burning
Friday	Turbocharged Fat Burning
Saturday	Calorie Restriction
Saturday night	Cheat Meal
Sunday	Carb Refuel

Weeks 5 and 6

Monday	Healthy Eating
Tuesday	Turbocharged Fat Burning
Wednesday	Turbocharged Fat Burning
Thursday	Turbocharged Fat Burning
Friday	Turbocharged Fat Burning
Saturday	Calorie Restriction
Saturday night	Cheat Meal
Sunday	Carb Refuel

Weeks 7 and 8

Monday	Turbocharged Fat Burning
Tuesday	Turbocharged Fat Burning
Wednesday	Turbocharged Fat Burning
Thursday	Turbocharged Fat Burning
Friday	Turbocharged Fat Burning
Saturday	Calorie Restriction
Saturday night	Cheat Meal
Sunday	Carb Refuel

MAINTENANCE PLAN

After 8 weeks on the Platinum 360 Nutrition Plan, you can continue to get great results by staying on the maintenance nutrition plan for as long as you want—even for the rest of your life. Just follow the same plan as you did during Weeks 1 and 2:

Monday	Healthy Eating
Tuesday	Healthy Eating
Wednesday	Healthy Eating
Thursday	Turbocharged Fat Burning
Friday	Turbocharged Fat Burning
Saturday	Calorie Restriction
Saturday night	Cheat Meal
Sunday	Carb Refuel

Healthy Eating: Moderate Carbs, Moderate Fat, High Protein

Purpose

The Healthy Eating plan keeps total calories fairly low while giving your body a balance of the nutrients it needs to function like a well-oiled machine. A big part of this strategy involves eating plenty of high-fiber, slow-digesting carbohydrates from fruits, vegetables, and whole grains. You'll be getting almost an equal amount of calories from carbs, fats, and protein. Long story short, you'll be taking in fewer calories than you're burning. Remember when I mentioned old-school math? Here it is at work. In total, you'll be getting almost an equal amount of calories from carbs, fats, and protein.

The Details

On Healthy Eating days, you'll keep your dietary fats and carbs moderate, emphasizing high-fiber, slow-digesting carbs such as oatmeal, brown rice, whole wheat pasta, sweet potatoes, fruits, and vegetables. Kick processed carbs to the curb (i.e., pasta, white bread, white potatoes, and anything that lists "refined wheat flour" or "enriched wheat flour" as the first ingredient). In total, your carb consumption should be about 1 gram for every pound you weigh. For fats, you'll emphasize unsaturated ones such as those from canola and olive oils, salmon and other fatty fish, nuts and seeds, and avocados. But you can also take in moderate amounts of saturated fats, particularly those that accompany good protein sources such as lean cuts of meat (beef, chicken, turkey, and fish) and dairy (milk, cheese, and eggs). Try to keep saturated fats to one-third of your total fat intake, with unsaturated fats making up the remaining two-thirds.

On Healthy Eating days, you'll also keep your protein intake fairly high—about 1 gram of protein per pound of body weight. While your calorie intake from carbs and protein is about the same, this is considered a "high protein" plan because most people typically eat far more carb than protein calories. The extra protein will help protect your muscle mass, providing amino acids for growth and recovery, and keep your metabolic rate up while keeping you satiated to prevent overeating, which enhances the burning of body fat. The moderate carbs will also help fuel activities so you won't feel depleted.

In all, you'll take in up to about 12 calories for every pound of body weight on Healthy Eating days. This low-to-moderate calorie intake helps you create a healthy calorie deficit. Coupled with an increase in activity through your workouts, your body will become a fat-burning machine.

By the Numbers

	Body Weight		
	Under 150	150–200	Over 200
Protein (g/cal)	140/560	170/680	200/800
Carbs (g/cal)	120/480	150/600	200/800
Fats (g/cal)	50/450	65/585	80/720
Total calories	1,490	1,865	2,320

HEALTHY EATING SAMPLE MEALS

While the meals included in this section add up to a daily plan that is moderate in carbs and dietary fats and high in protein, the macronutrients shift a bit from one meal to another because your body has different needs at different times of the day. For instance, you eat no fat before your workouts, and you eat no carbs before you go to bed.

Healthy Eating Breakfasts

For breakfast, you want to emphasize protein and slow-digesting carbs. Protein helps refeed your muscles after they've gone several hours without food while you were sleeping, and slow-digesting carbs give you long-lasting fuel that will remain available for a few hours, so you will be energetic throughout your morning activities and keep your body burning fat throughout the day.

Protein shake and English muffin

	Under 150 lbs	150–200 lbs	Over 200 lbs
Whey protein	1 scoop (mix in 1 cup water)	1 scoop	1½ scoops
Whole wheat English muffin	½	1	1
Low-sugar preserves	1 Tbsp	1 Tbsp	1 Tbsp

Scrambled eggs with cheese and waffle with fruit

	Under 150 lbs	150–200 lbs	Over 200 lbs
Large egg	1	1	2
Large egg whites	2	3	3
Low-fat American cheese	1 slice	1 slice	1 slice
Low-fat whole grain waffle (such as Van's)	1	2	2
Sliced strawberries	¼ cup	½ cup	½ cup

Breakfast sandwich and side of cottage cheese

	Under 150 lbs	150–200 lbs	Over 200 lbs
Large egg (fried in nonstick cooking spray)	1	1	2
Low-fat cheese	1 slice	1 slice	1 slice
Whole wheat English muffin	1	1	1
Cottage cheese	¼ cup	½ cup	½ cup

Scrambled eggs with cheese and peanut butter banana

	Under 150 lbs	150–200 lbs	Over 200 lbs
Large egg	1	1	2
Large egg whites	2	3	3
Low-fat American cheese	1 slice	1 slice	1 slice
Large banana	½	½	1
Peanut butter	1 Tbsp	1 Tbsp	1 Tbsp

Cottage cheese with pineapple and fruit-topped waffle

	Under 150 lbs	150–200 lbs	Over 200 lbs
Low-fat cottage cheese	¼ cup	¾ cup	1 cup
Diced pineapple	¼ cup	¼ cup	¼ cup
Low-fat whole grain waffle (such as Van's)	1	1	1
Sliced strawberries	¼ cup	½ cup	½ cup

Scrambled eggs and oatmeal

	Under 150 lbs	150–200 lbs	Over 200 lbs
Large egg	1	1	2
Large egg whites	2	3	3
Low-fat American cheese	1 slice	1 slice	1 slice
Plain oatmeal	½ cup cooked	1 cup cooked	1 cup cooked

Add noncaloric sweetener and cinnamon to taste.

Healthy Eating Late-Morning Snacks

After you've been awake for a few hours, you may notice that you're starting to feel a little hungry as your breakfast empties from your stomach. At this point, you want to eat another meal that's high in protein, with just a moderate amount of fats and carbs. You don't need a lot of calories because your lunch is not far off.

Cottage cheese and fruit

	Under 150 lbs	150–200 lbs	Over 200 lbs
Low-fat cottage cheese	¼ cup	½ cup	¾ cup
Diced pineapple	¼ cup	¼ cup	¼ cup

You may substitute ½ cup of any kind of sliced fruit, blueberries, or other berries for the pineapple.

Steak and edamame

	Under 150 lbs	150–200 lbs	Over 200 lbs
Top sirloin	2–3 oz	4 oz	5–6 oz
Edamame	¼ cup	½ cup	½ cup

Shrimp cocktail with veggies

	Under 150 lbs	150–200 lbs	Over 200 lbs
Boiled shrimp	2–3 oz	4 oz	4–6 oz
Cocktail sauce	1 Tbsp	1 Tbsp	1 Tbsp
Steamed veggies	½ cup	1 cup	1 cup

Healthy Eating Lunches

These lunch options are high in protein, with moderate amounts of slow-digesting carbs and dietary fats. It's important to keep feeding your body every 2 to 3 hours so that you have a constant supply of energy and amino acids circulating through your system. This prevents you from feeling hungry and keeps your metabolism up, especially on workout days, when you'll have a greater need for energy and nutrients.

Deli sandwich

	Under 150 lbs	150–200 lbs	Over 200 lbs
Sliced deli roast beef or turkey	3 oz	4 oz	4–6 oz
Low-fat cheese	1 slice	1 slice	1 slice
Whole wheat bread	1 slice	2 slices	2 slices
Fat-free mayonnaise	1 Tbsp	1 Tbsp	1 Tbsp

Lean burger and veggies

	Under 150 lbs	150–200 lbs	Over 200 lbs
95% lean beef patty or turkey burger	3 oz	4 oz	6–8 oz
Low-fat cheese (optional)	1 slice	1 slice	1 slice
Whole wheat hamburger bun	1	1	1
Ketchup (optional)	1 Tbsp	1 Tbsp	1 Tbsp
Steamed Brussels sprouts	1 cup	1 cup	1 cup

Tuna pita and veggies

	Under 150 lbs	150–200 lbs	Over 200 lbs
Light tuna in water	½ can	½ can	1 can
Low-fat mayonnaise	1 Tbsp	1 Tbsp	1 Tbsp
Whole wheat pita	1 medium	1 large	1 large
Steamed asparagus	1 cup	1 cup	1 cup

Spaghetti with meatballs

	Under 150 lbs	150–200 lbs	Over 200 lbs
Ground turkey or lean beef meatballs (page 204)	4 oz	4 oz	6–8 oz
Whole wheat pasta	½ cup	1 cup	1 cup
Low-fat marinara sauce	⅛ cup	¼ cup	¼ cup

Shrimp and beans on rice

	Under 150 lbs	150–200 lbs	Over 200 lbs
Boiled shrimp	4 oz	4 oz	6–8 oz
Cooked brown rice	¼ cup	½ cup	½ cup
Cooked black beans	¼ cup	½ cup	½ cup

Mediterranean fish pocket

	Under 150 lbs	150–200 lbs	Over 200 lbs
Baked tilapia or sole	4 oz	4 oz	6–8 oz
Whole wheat pita	1 medium	1 large	1 large
Hummus	⅛ cup	¼ cup	¼ cup
Lettuce leaves and/or hot sauce			

Chicken salad in pita

	Under 150 lbs	150–200 lbs	Over 200 lbs
Cooked chicken breast	3 oz	3 oz	6 oz
Low-fat mayonnaise	1 Tbsp	1 Tbsp	1 Tbsp
Whole wheat pita	1 medium	1 large	1 large
Raspberries	½ cup	1 cup	1 cup

Healthy Eating Midday Snacks

Halfway between lunch and dinner, you should eat a midday snack that is low in fat, with moderate carbs.

Fruit and yogurt

	Under 150 lbs	150–200 lbs	Over 200 lbs
Low-fat plain yogurt	6 oz	8 oz	10 oz
Blueberries (or other fruit or berries)	¼ cup	½ cup	½ cup

Fish with soup

	Under 150 lbs	150–200 lbs	Over 200 lbs
Baked tilapia or sole	2–3 oz	4 oz	4–6 oz
Tomato soup	½ cup	1 cup	1 cup

Tuna on crackers

	Under 150 lbs	150–200 lbs	Over 200 lbs
Tuna fish in water	¼ can	½ can	½ can
Low-fat mayo	<1 Tbsp	1 Tbsp	1 Tbsp
Whole wheat crackers (such as Ak-Mak)	3	4	6

Pre- or postworkout special: protein shake and fruit

	Under 150 lbs	150–200 lbs	Over 200 lbs
Whey protein	¾ scoop	1 scoop	1½ scoops
Peaches	1 medium	1 large	2 medium

Healthy Eating Dinners

Dinner provides a few more calories than the other meals of the day and emphasizes protein, with a relatively small amount of slow-digesting carbs. As you get toward the end of the day, your need for carb energy, especially from fast-digesting carbs, decreases because your activity levels also go down. The fats further slow your digestive rate.

Shrimp and rice stir-fry

	Under 150 lbs	150–200 lbs	Over 200 lbs
Raw fresh shrimp	4 oz	4 oz	6–8 oz
Medium onion, sliced	¼	½	½
Bean sprouts	¼ cup	¼ cup	¼ cup
Peas	¼ cup	¼ cup	¼ cup
Brown rice	½ cup	1 cup	1 cup

Coat a skillet with cooking spray, stir-fry onion and sprouts, then add shrimp and peas and toss until cooked through. Serve over brown rice.

Fish, rice, and green beans

	Under 150 lbs	150–200 lbs	Over 200 lbs
Baked tilapia or sole	4 oz	4 oz	6–8 oz
Cooked brown rice	½ cup	¾ cup	1 cup
Steamed green beans	½ cup	½ cup	½ cup

Chicken broccoli pizza

Food	Under 150 lbs	150–200 lbs	Over 200 lbs
8" whole wheat pizza crust	⅛	⅛	¼
Fat-free shredded mozzarella	¼ cup	¼ cup	½ cup
Tomato sauce	2 Tbsp	2 Tbsp	3 Tbsp
Diced cooked chicken breast	3 oz	4 oz	4–6 oz
Chopped broccoli	½ cup	½ cup	½ cup

Spaghetti and meatballs

	Under 150 lbs	150–200 lbs	Over 200 lbs
Ground turkey or lean beef meatballs (page 204)	4 oz	4 oz	6–8 oz
Cooked soba noodles	½ cup	1 cup	1 cup
Marinara sauce	⅛ cup	¼ cup	¼ cup

Tilapia with quinoa and veggies

	Under 150 lbs	150–200 lbs	Over 200 lbs
Baked tilapia	4 oz	4 oz	6–8 oz
Cooked quinoa	½ cup	¾ cup	1 cup
Steamed zucchini or broccoli	½ cup	½ cup	½ cup

Spelt salad with shrimp and green beans

	Under 150 lbs	150–200 lbs	Over 200 lbs
Steamed shrimp	4 oz	4 oz	6–8 oz
Cooked spelt	¼ cup	½ cup	1 cup
Green beans	½ cup	½ cup	½ cup

Chopped herbs or lemon juice to taste.

Shrimp or chicken quesadilla

	Under 150 lbs	150–200 lbs	Over 200 lbs
Cooked shrimp or diced chicken	3 oz	4 oz	4–6 oz
Low-fat or fat-free shredded cheese	⅛ cup	⅛ cup	¼ cup
Whole wheat tortilla	1 medium	1 large	2 medium
Tomato salsa	2 Tbsp	2 Tbsp	¼ cup

Chicken dinner

	Under 150 lbs	150–200 lbs	Over 200 lbs
Chicken breast	6 oz	6 oz	8 oz
Baked sweet potato	1 small	1 medium	1 large
Steamed chopped broccoli	1 cup	1 cup	1 cup
Salad greens	1 cup	2 cups	2 cups
Salad dressing (olive oil and vinegar)	1 Tbsp	1½ Tbsp	2 Tbsp

Healthy Eating Nighttime Snacks

Refuel one more time before you hit the sack, but stay away from carbs that will sit in your stomach during your most inactive period.

Hard-boiled egg

	Under 150 lbs	150–200 lbs	Over 200 lbs
Hard-boiled eggs	2 medium	2 large	2 extra large

Mixed Nuts

	Under 150 lbs	150–200 lbs	Over 200 lbs
Mixed nuts	1 oz	1 oz	1½ oz

Low-fat cheese

	Under 150 lbs	150–200 lbs	Over 200 lbs
Low-fat cheese	1½ oz	2 oz	2½ oz

Protein shake

	Under 150 lbs	150–200 lbs	Over 200 lbs
Whey protein	¾ scoop	1 scoop	1½ scoops

Turbocharged Fat Burning: Low Carbs, High Fat, High Protein

Purpose

To get your body's fat-burning potential revved up to its highest level, you want to reduce and replace some, though not all, of these calories with dietary fats. Your body will release less insulin, encouraging your body to pull more fat from storage. On Turbocharged Fat Burning days, you'll be creating an even larger calorie deficit. Keep protein high, and you can take it up a little bit more than on Healthy Eating days. If you find it simply isn't enough food for you, you can increase the amount of protein a bit. Just don't add more carbs.

The Details

When you're turbocharging your diet, you'll eat only about ½ gram of carbs for every pound of body weight. This means that a woman under 150 pounds will consume no more than 60 grams of carbs a day, someone between 150 and 200 pounds will consume no more than about 70 to 90 grams of carbs, and a man who weighs 200 or more pounds will consume no more than 100 grams of carbs on each of these days. Without many carbs to burn, your body will turn to stored fat for fuel. In addition, most of the carbs you consume will come from slow-digesting carbs (fruits, vegetables, and whole grains), and you'll take most of these in early in the day, cutting back in the afternoon and at dinner.

While you're restricting carbs, you can eat foods that have a little more fat, especially healthy unsaturated ones, like salads dressed with oil and vinegar, some sliced avocado on your chicken lettuce wrap, or baked or grilled fatty fish like salmon. You can also continue to take in saturated fats with whole foods such as lean meats, cheese, and eggs. Keep in mind that many forms of dairy, such as milk and yogurt, have carbs in addition to protein, so it's best to steer clear or at least drastically reduce consumption of these foods when you're cutting carbs. In total, aim for about 60 grams of fat a day if you weigh less than 150 pounds, about 70 to 80 grams if you weigh between 150 to 200 pounds, and up to about 90 grams of fat if you weigh more than 200 pounds.

Meanwhile, keep taking in that protein. While my "By the Numbers" chart shows that you should consume the same amount of protein as you do during your Healthy Eating phase, you may find the need to add a little more protein to your plan to keep you from feeling hungry. On the other hand, many people find that because the meals are already high in protein, which takes longer to digest (keeping you feeling fuller), the plan provides plenty of food, actually making it difficult to consume the recommended amount of food in 1 day, even across six meals. Again, this high-protein intake will help protect your body from burning muscle mass.

In total, you should take in about 10 to 11 calories for every pound of body weight.

By the Numbers

	Body Weight		
	Under 150	150–200	Over 200
Protein (g/cal)	140/560	170/680	200/800
Carbs (g/cal)	60/240	80/320	100/400
Fats (g/cal)	60/540	75/675	90/810
Total calories	1,340	1,675	2,010

TURBOCHARGED FAT BURNING SAMPLE MEALS

The meals in this section make up a daily plan that is low in carbs, high in fats, and high in protein. As with Healthy Eating, the macronutrients shift throughout the day: You'll eat fewer carbs in the second half of the day than you did at the beginning.

Pick from the meal options provided or use them as a model to design similar meal options. You can also choose from any of the recipes for Turbocharged Fat Burning in the next chapter to create your own meal plans. No one says you had to stop getting creative to start eating right.

Turbocharged Fat Burning Breakfasts

Turbocharged Fat Burning breakfasts contain a few less carbs than those in the Healthy Eating section, but the calories are basically the same. You do need some carbs to fuel activities through the day, but reducing them also helps you burn more stored body fat. For breakfast, you replace some carb calories with fats and protein.

Scrambled eggs with cheese and oatmeal

	Under 150 lbs	150–200 lbs	Over 200 lbs
Eggs	2 medium	2 large	2 jumbo
Egg whites	2 medium	2 large	2 jumbo
Low-fat American cheese	1 slice	1 slice	1 slice
Oatmeal with noncaloric sweetener and cinnamon to taste	½ cup	½ cup	¾ cup

Protein shake and English muffin with preserves

	Under 150 lbs	150–200 lbs	Over 200 lbs
Whey protein	1 scoop	1½ scoops	2 scoops
Whole wheat English muffin	½	½	1
Low-sugar preserves	1 Tbsp	1 Tbsp	1 Tbsp

Cottage cheese with pineapple

	Under 150 lbs	150–200 lbs	Over 200 lbs
Low-fat cottage cheese	¾ cup	¾ cup	1 cup
Diced pineapple	¼ cup	½ cup	¾ cup

Scrambled eggs with cheese and waffle with fruit

	Under 150 lbs	150–200 lbs	Over 200 lbs
Eggs	2 medium	2 large	2 jumbo
Egg whites	2 medium	2 large	2 jumbo
Low-fat American cheese	1 slice	1 slice	1 slice
Low-fat whole grain waffle (such as Van's)	½	1	1½
Sliced strawberries	¼ cup	¼ cup	¼ cup

Egg and cheese sandwich

	Under 150 lbs	150–200 lbs	Over 200 lbs
Eggs (fried)	2 medium	2 large	2 jumbo
Low-fat American cheese (optional)	1 slice	1 slice	1 slice
Whole wheat English muffin	½	1	1½
Low-fat cottage cheese	¼ cup	¼ cup	½ cup

Scrambled eggs with cheese and peanut butter banana

	Under 150 lbs	150–200 lbs	Over 200 lbs
Eggs	2 medium	2 large	2 jumbo
Egg whites	2 medium	2 large	2 jumbo
Low-fat American cheese	1 slice	1 slice	1 slice
Banana	½ small	½ large	1 large
Peanut butter	1 Tbsp	1 Tbsp	1 Tbsp

Cottage cheese with pineapple and waffle with fruit

	Under 150 lbs	150–200 lbs	Over 200 lbs
Low-fat cottage cheese	½ cup	¾ cup	1 cup
Diced pineapple	¼ cup	¼ cup	¼ cup
Low-fat whole grain waffle (such as Van's)	½	1	1½
Sliced strawberries	¼ cup	¼ cup	¼ cup

Scrambled eggs and cereal

	Under 150 lbs	150–200 lbs	Over 200 lbs
Eggs	2 medium	2 large	2 jumbo
Egg whites	2 medium	2 large	2 jumbo
High-fiber cereal (no sugar added)	⅓ cup	½ cup	¾ cup
Low-fat milk	2 oz	3 oz	4 oz

Turbocharged Fat Burning Late-Morning Snacks

Late-morning snacks on your Turbocharged Fat Burning days generally contain a few carbs to continue to provide fuel that will stay with you for a few hours. These snacks also contain protein and fats to satisfy your cravings so you won't get hungry before lunch.

Cottage cheese with fruit

	Under 150 lbs	150–200 lbs	Over 200 lbs
Low-fat cottage cheese	½ cup	¾ cup	1 cup
Diced pineapple	¼ cup	¼ cup	½ cup

You may substitute ¼ cup of any kind of sliced fruit, blueberries, or other berries for the pineapple.

Steak and edamame

	Under 150 lbs	150–200 lbs	Over 200 lbs
Top sirloin	2 oz	3 oz	4 oz
Edamame	¼ cup	¼ cup	½ cup

Shrimp cocktail with veggies

	Under 150 lbs	150–200 lbs	Over 200 lbs
Cooked shrimp	2 oz	3 oz	4 oz
Seafood cocktail sauce	1 Tbsp	1 Tbsp	1 Tbsp
Mixed veggies	½ cup	½ cup	½ cup

Grilled fish and soup

	Under 150 lbs	150–200 lbs	Over 200 lbs
Salmon, tilapia, or sole	2 oz	3 oz	4 oz
Tomato soup	⅓ cup	½ cup	¾ cup

Turbocharged Fat Burning Lunches

These lunches are relatively low in calories and very low in carbs, a real change from the Healthy Eating meal options. Consequently, they contain a bit more fat, so you can continue to provide your body with a steady stream of amino acids, helping to ensure that your muscle won't be broken down for other processes. On the other hand, you may begin to feel a little depleted on your Turbocharged Fat Burning phase. You shouldn't be overly hungry, but you may find you don't have as much energy during your weight workouts. Take that in stride. That means that the program is working—you're tapping into body fat for fuel while you're protecting your muscles with plenty of protein.

Beef, cheese, and avocado

	Under 150 lbs	150–200 lbs	Over 200 lbs
Roast beef	3 oz	4 oz	5–6 oz
Low-fat American cheese	3 slices	4 slices	5 slices
Avocado	½ medium	½ medium	¾ medium

Veggies with cottage cheese dip

	Under 150 lbs	150–200 lbs	Over 200 lbs
Low-fat cottage cheese	½ cup	½ cup	¾ cup
Shelled sunflower seeds	¾ Tbsp	1 Tbsp	1¼ Tbsp
Celery and green peppers	1 cup	1 cup	1 cup

Mix seeds in cottage cheese; use as a dip for the vegetables.

Protein shake and mixed nuts

	Under 150 lbs	150–200 lbs	Over 200 lbs
Whey protein	1 scoop	1 scoop	1½ scoops
Mixed nuts	¾ oz	1 oz	1½ oz

Steak and eggs

	Under 150 lbs	150–200 lbs	Over 200 lbs
Steak	3 oz	4 oz	5 oz
Eggs	1 medium	1 large	2 medium

Turkey-and-cheese lettuce wrap with veggies

	Under 150 lbs	150–200 lbs	Over 200 lbs
Turkey deli meat	4 oz	4–6 oz	6 oz
Low-fat cheese *(optional)*	1 slice	1 slice	1 slice
Low-fat mayo or mustard	1 Tbsp	1 Tbsp	1 Tbsp
Mixed vegetables	½ cup	½ cup	½ cup
Romaine lettuce leaf	1 large	1 large	1 large

Wrap turkey, cheese, and mayo in lettuce.

Tuna-salad lettuce wrap

	Under 150 lbs	150–200 lbs	Over 200 lbs
Light tuna (in water)	¾ can	¾ can	1 can
Low-fat mayo	1 Tbsp	1½ Tbsp	2 Tbsp
Chopped medium onion	¼	¼	¼
Chopped celery	1 rib	1 rib	1 rib
Romaine lettuce leaf	1 large	1 large	1 large

Mix tuna, mayo, onion, and celery; wrap in lettuce.

Chicken, avocado, and veggie wraps

	Under 150 lbs	150–200 lbs	Over 200 lbs
Chicken breast	4 oz	6 oz	8 oz
Avocado	¼	¼	½
Chopped raw veggies	2 oz	2 oz	2 oz
Romaine lettuce leaf	1 large	1 large	1 large

Turbocharged Fat Burning Midday Snacks

It's important to give yourself a snack midway between lunch and dinner, especially when you're following a low-carb plan. Some additional fuel in the form of (mostly) protein and fats is the best way to make sure you don't feel hungry or sluggish.

Celery with peanut butter

	Under 150 lbs	150–200 lbs	Over 200 lbs
Celery	2 ribs	2 ribs	2 ribs
Peanut butter	1 Tbsp	1 Tbsp	1 Tbsp

Canned sardines

	Under 150 lbs	150–200 lbs	Over 200 lbs
Sardines in water or mustard	½ tin	¾ tin	1 tin

Deli roll-ups

	Under 150 lbs	150–200 lbs	Over 200 lbs
Lean deli meat	2 oz	3 oz	4 oz
Low-fat mozzarella cheese	1 oz	2 oz	2 oz

Protein shake

	Under 150 lbs	150–200 lbs	Over 200 lbs
Whey protein	1 scoop	1½ scoops	2 scoops

Turbocharged Fat Burning Dinners

Dinner provides more calories than the other meals of the day, without a corresponding jump in the carb count. When you're restricting carbs, it's even more critical to watch your intake during the second half of the day, when your energy needs are reduced. These meals also include a healthy amount of fats to provide satiety and keep your metabolic rate revved up.

Salmon, bok choy, and salad

	Under 150 lbs	150–200 lbs	Over 200 lbs
Salmon	5 oz	6 oz	8 oz
Steamed bok choy	1 cup	1 cup	1 cup
Salad greens	1½ cups	2 cups	2½ cups
Salad dressing (olive oil and vinegar)	1½ Tbsp	2 Tbsp	2½ Tbsp

Tilapia, asparagus, and salad

	Under 150 lbs	150–200 lbs	Over 200 lbs
Cooked tilapia	6 oz	8 oz	10 oz
Asparagus	1 cup	1 cup	1 cup
Salad greens	1½ cups	2 cups	2½ cups
Salad dressing (olive oil and vinegar)	1½ Tbsp	2 Tbsp	2½ Tbsp

Bunless burger with fixin's

	Under 150 lbs	150–200 lbs	Over 200 lbs
95% lean hamburger	6 oz	8 oz	10 oz
Onion	1 slice	1 slice	1 slice
Tomato	1 slice	1 slice	1 slice
Romaine lettuce wrapper	1 large	1 large	1 large
Low-fat mayo and/or mustard	1 Tbsp	1 Tbsp	1 Tbsp

Shrimp cocktail and green beans sautéed in olive oil

	Under 150 lbs	150–200 lbs	Over 200 lbs
Cooked shrimp	6 oz	8 oz	10 oz
Cocktail sauce	1 Tbsp	1 Tbsp	1 Tbsp
Green beans	1 cup	1 cup	1 cup
Olive oil	1½ Tbsp	2 Tbsp	2 Tbsp

Chicken and avocado salad

	Under 150 lbs	150–200 lbs	Over 200 lbs
Chicken breast	6 oz	8 oz	10 oz
Avocado	¼ medium	¼ medium	¼ medium
Salad greens	1½ cups	2 cups	2½ cups
Salad dressing (olive oil and vinegar)	1½ Tbsp	2 Tbsp	2½ Tbsp

Pork roast

	Under 150 lbs	150–200 lbs	Over 200 lbs
Pork roast	4 oz	6 oz	8 oz
Onion	½	½	½
Celery	2 ribs	3 ribs	4 ribs

Roast pork with onions and celery. Pork should reach an internal temperature of 155° to 160°F, letting the onions and celery absorb some of the fat if you want. Pat dry before eating to reduce calories.

Turbocharged Fat Burning Nighttime Snack

During this phase, you want to consume some protein and fats to feed your body throughout the night, but continue to avoid carbs.

Cottage cheese with salsa

	Under 150 lbs	150–200 lbs	Over 200 lbs
Low-fat cottage cheese	½ cup	½ cup	½ cup
Salsa	¼ cup	¼ cup	¼ cup

Canned sardines

	Under 150 lbs	150–200 lbs	Over 200 lbs
Sardines in water or mustard	½ tin	¾ tin	1 tin

Hard-boiled eggs

	Under 150 lbs	150–200 lbs	Over 200 lbs
Hard-boiled eggs	2 medium	2 large	2 jumbo

Turkey avocado roll-ups

	Under 150 lbs	150–200 lbs	Over 200 lbs
Sliced turkey breast	2 oz	3 oz	4 oz
Avocado	1 slice	2 slices	3 slices

Calorie Restriction: No Carbs, Low Fat, High Protein

Purpose

These meals deplete your body of both carbs and fat in preparation for the huge influx you'll be getting from your Cheat Meal later in the day. While extreme calorie cutting can have negative effects on your metabolic rate, that's not the case on this plan because this phase lasts less than 24 hours—from your bedtime snack the night before to your dinner the next night. Your body will be drained and ready for fuel by the time your reward Cheat Meal rolls around on Saturday night. When you refeed, it will taste great, but it will do wonders to restore your glycogen stocks, rev up your metabolism, and, most important, make certain that you continue to get great results.

The Details

A day of denial probably sounds tough, and sometimes it is. Just keep reminding yourself you only have to make it to 6:00 or 7:00 p.m. Better still, when you do make it, you'll get to eat whatever you want and go to bed well fed.

You may be wondering about the point of eating virtually no carbs from the night before (Friday) until your Cheat Meal on Saturday evening. Think of it this way: Your muscles act somewhat like sponges. The less water a sponge contains, the more it is able to absorb. With muscles, the less glycogen that is stored in them, the more glycogen they are able to take in when nutrients (especially carbs) are introduced into the bloodstream. Going no-carb is akin to wringing all the glycogen out of your muscles.

On your Calorie Restriction plan, you must avoid all carbs—even in the form of condi-ments. Concentrate almost exclusively on foods that contain protein and a little fat. You'll also eat considerably fewer calories during the day because (1) it's hard to get in a lot of calories if all you're eating is protein and some fats and (2) you want to control your intake so that you don't consume too many calories before your Cheat Meal in the evening.

During the Calorie Restriction phase, you'll eat only four meals, as opposed to the usual five on my plan: breakfast, a late-morning snack, lunch, and a midday snack. Each of these meals will be fairly small, in the 100-calorie to 300-calorie range, depending on the meal and your body weight. (Check out the chart below to see just how few calories you'll be taking in for the first two-thirds of your day.) By the time you reach your evening Cheat Meal, you'll be in a major calorie deficit for the day, but don't worry—that meal will more than make up for what you passed up during the day.

One thing you may have noticed is that your Saturday Calorie Restriction strategy followed by the Cheat Meal remains consistent throughout the 8 weeks of the Platinum 360 Nutrition Plan. While your Healthy Eating and Turbocharged Fat Burning strategies shift every 2 weeks throughout the 8-week plan, these brief—but extremely crucial—phases remain a constant. These combined strategies are a great way to spike your metabolism and encourage fat burning and muscle building.

By the Numbers

	Body Weight		
	Under 150	150–200	Over 200
Protein (g/cal)	80/320	100/400	120/480
Carbs (g/cal)	0/0	0/0	0/0
Fats (g/cal)	25/225	30/270	40/360
Total calories	545	670	840

Values do not include the Cheat Meal.

Calorie Restriction Sample Meals

The goal is to deplete—almost thoroughly—your glycogen stores. You'll still provide your body with small amounts of fuel, but it will be in the form of protein and fat. Don't be surprised if you don't feel as energetic as you normally do when you have carbs in your bloodstream throughout the day.

The meals in this section contain very few to no carbs. It's important that you not only eat moderate to small amounts of protein and fats but also cut out carbs almost completely. This temporary deprivation is what provides the dramatic metabolic boost when you refeed later in the day.

Calorie Restriction Breakfasts

This is the kickoff to your no-carb day. Breakfast will be tasty. You'll eat eggs, breakfast meat, cheese, and other protein/fat sources. This meal will satisfy your hunger without really refueling you because it contains no carbs. Hold tight; that's coming later in the day.

Scrambled eggs with cheese

	Under 150 lbs	150–200 lbs	Over 200 lbs
Eggs	2 medium	2 large	2 jumbo
Egg whites	2 medium	2 large	2 jumbo
Low-fat American cheese	1 slice	1 slice	1 slice

Scrambled eggs with chicken sausage

	Under 150 lbs	150–200 lbs	Over 200 lbs
Low-fat chicken sausage	2 links	3 links	4 links
Egg	1 medium	1 large	1 jumbo
Egg whites	2 large	3 large	4 large

Steak and eggs

	Under 150 lbs	150–200 lbs	Over 200 lbs
Breakfast steak	4 oz	5 oz	6 oz
Egg	1 medium	1 large	1 jumbo

Turkey omelet

	Under 150 lbs	150–200 lbs	Over 200 lbs
Eggs	2 medium	2 large	2 jumbo
Turkey deli meat	1 oz	2 oz	3 oz

Calorie Restriction Late-Morning Snacks

When you're eating only protein and carbs, you're going to get hungry, so making one of these snacks will help you get through your no-carb Saturdays. They may be small, but they're an essential part of making sure that you don't get *over*depleted.

Cottage cheese

	Under 150 lbs	150–200 lbs	Over 200 lbs
Low-fat cottage cheese	⅓ cup	½ cup	¾ cup

Deli meat

	Under 150 lbs	150–200 lbs	Over 200 lbs
Low-fat turkey or ham	4 oz	6 oz	8 oz

Nuts

	Under 150 lbs	150–200 lbs	Over 200 lbs
Almonds	2 Tbsp	3 Tbsp	4 Tbsp

Calorie Restriction Lunches

All these lunches are high in protein and contain a reasonable amount of dietary fats. Considering how low in calories they are, they will stay with you for a fairly long time, so you'll be eating very low calorie, but you won't be hungry.

Beef, cheese, and avocado roll-ups

	Under 150 lbs	150–200 lbs	Over 200 lbs
Roast beef	3 oz	4 oz	5 oz
Low-fat American cheese	3 slices	4 slices	4 slices
Avocado	⅓	½	¾

Bunless cheeseburger

	Under 150 lbs	150–200 lbs	Over 200 lbs
95% lean hamburger meat	5 oz	6 oz	8 oz
Low-fat cheese	1 slice	1 slice	1 slice

Chicken, cheese, and avocado

	Under 150 lbs	150–200 lbs	Over 200 lbs
Chicken breast	5 oz	6 oz	8 oz
Low-fat American cheese	1 slice	2 slices	3 slices
Avocado	⅓	½	¾

Turkey, egg, and avocado roll-ups

	Under 150 lbs	150–200 lbs	Over 200 lbs
Turkey deli slices	4 oz	6 oz	8 oz
Hard-boiled egg	1 medium	1 large	1 jumbo
Avocado	1 slice	2 slices	3 slices

Calorie Restriction Midday Snacks

At this point in the day, you don't need a lot of calories, just a little sustenance in the form of protein and fats to get through the next few hours before your payoff dinner. The small number of calories in these midday snacks is derived almost entirely from protein and fats.

Celery with peanut butter

	Under 150 lbs	150–200 lbs	Over 200 lbs
Celery	2 ribs	2 ribs	3 ribs
Peanut butter	1 Tbsp	1 Tbsp	1½ Tbsp

Canned sardines

	Under 150 lbs	150–200 lbs	Over 200 lbs
Sardines in water or mustard	½ tin	¾ tin	1 tin

Cottage cheese

	Under 150 lbs	150–200 lbs	Over 200 lbs
Low-fat cottage cheese	½ cup	¾ cup	1 cup

Nuts

	Under 150 lbs	150–200 lbs	Over 200 lbs
Walnuts	1½ oz	2 oz	2½ oz

Cheat Meal: High Carbs, High Fats, Moderate Protein

Purpose

You've made it! This meal is your reward for sticking to the plan all week long. Choose your poison: pizza and beer, chili cheese fries, a loaded cheeseburger—you name it. They're all fair game after the regimen you've followed over the past 24 hours in preparation. The only caveat is you must keep total calories in check; don't gorge yourself and undo all the good you did earlier in the week. (Check out the "By the Numbers" chart to make sure that you aren't overdoing it.)

The Details

It may seem like the Cheat Meal will undercut all the sweat and sacrifices you've endured for the previous 6 days, but on the contrary, this meal is an important part of the program. A large influx of calories, taken in irregularly, provides a major metabolic boost. If you cut your calories too low and never exceed that bottom-basement level, you send your body the message that it needs to hoard body fat. By providing a large influx of calories every once in a while, you calm down the warning signs your body receives from long-term calorie deprivation.

Here's another way to look at it: By dieting rigorously throughout the week and monitoring your macronutrients, you've trained your body for endurance. Providing a huge influx of calories is akin to telling your body that it's now ready for strength. This is the start of your refeed phase, to be followed by your Carb Refuel on Sunday. Between these two, you reassure your body that it is not going through a period of starvation, allowing it to continue to shed the fat reserves it has been storing for a rainy day.

So, *how much can you eat?* Check out the "By the Numbers" chart below, which will give you guidelines on how to refeed yourself without gorging.

By the Numbers

	Body Weight		
	Under 150	150–200	Over 200
Protein (g/cal)	40/160	50/200	60/240
Carbs (g/cal)	125/500	175/700	225/900
Fats (g/cal)	30/270	40/360	50/450
Total calories	930	1,260	1,590

Values are for Cheat Meal only.

Note that you can eat any food that you want during your Cheat Meal, but try to consume a reasonable amount of protein (about 30 to 40 grams). Love burgers? Great—they have protein. So does pizza. Alcohol doesn't, so add some cheese or meat to the mix. And keep calories within reason for your body weight—approximately 7 to 8 calories for every pound of body weight.

Carb Refuel: High Carbs, Low Fat, High Protein

Purpose

Continue reloading your glycogen stores, the process you started the night before with your Cheat Meal. By taking in more carbs, you provide your body with a store to hold in your muscle tissue until you use it for your workouts during the upcoming week. This will not only rev up your metabolic rate, it will provide you with energy, particularly during your workouts.

The Details

On Sundays, you'll eat significantly more carbs than at any other time of the week. This is the day where you can satisfy your craving for all those sugary and starchy foods that you cut from your plan the rest of the week. This includes white rice, jelly beans, angel food cake, pancakes with syrup—anything that's high in carbs and low in fat. On Sundays, you may consume around 2 grams of carbs for every pound of body weight. A person who weighs less than 150 pounds should consume up to about 240 grams of carbs, and a person who weighs more than 200 pounds should consume up to about 400 grams of carbs on this day.

You'll keep your protein intake high—about 1 gram of protein for every pound of body weight. On the other hand, you'll be cutting your intake of fat significantly—only about 10 percent of your calories should come from fats on high-carb days. A person who weighs less than 150 pounds should take in only up to about 20 grams of fat, and a person who weighs more than 200 pounds should try to keep fat intake to no more than about 30 grams. Keep in mind that many protein foods also contain fats, and you should emphasize leaner sources of protein on Sundays. Foods such as most pork products, all but the leanest cuts of beef, dairy (except fat-free and low-fat varieties), and whole eggs contain dietary fats that may take you above your allotted amount for the day if you don't watch the quantities and the numbers on the foods that you're eating.

The good news is that you can eat any type of carbs you want, and you can eat them throughout the day to provide your body with stored energy for the week ahead. Both fast- and slow-digesting carbs can help with this. The problem with storing carbs as body fat comes from eating fast-digesting carbs too frequently when you don't need them. While slow-digesting carbs may be a better option, you've been deprived of fast-digesting carbs such as sugar and starchy carbs throughout the week, so now is a good time to enjoy them. These types of carbs can help keep your metabolic rate up, which means you keep dropping body fat. Too many diets limit carbs for too long. This can lead to a drop in metabolic rate and a halt in your progress. On the 360 Platinum Nutrition Plan, the Carb Refuel prevents this from happening.

By the Numbers

	Body Weight		
	Under 150	150–200	Over 200
Protein (g/cal)	140/560	170/680	200/800
Carbs (g/cal)	240/960	320/1,280	400/1,600
Fats (g/cal)	20/180	25/225	30/270
Total calories	1,700	2,185	2,670

Carb Refuel Breakfasts

You may already feel robust and refueled from your Cheat Meal the night before, but don't overlook the importance of getting in carbs from the start to the end of the day on Sunday. These carbs will provide your body with fuel that will take you a few days into the next week, helping to provide you with energy during the lower-carb phase that's coming around again. Note that high-carb breakfasts are very low in fat, compared with other days of the week.

Scrambled eggs with cheese and waffle with syrup

	Under 150 lbs	150–200 lbs	Over 200 lbs
Egg	1 medium	1 large	1 jumbo
Egg whites	2 large	3 large	4 large
Low-fat American cheese	1 slice	1 slice	1 slice
Low-fat whole grain waffle (such as Van's)	1	1	1½
Maple syrup	½ Tbsp	1 Tbsp	1½ Tbsp

Scrambled eggs and pancakes

	Under 150 lbs	150–200 lbs	Over 200 lbs
Egg	1 medium	1 large	1 jumbo
Egg whites	2 large	3 large	4 large
Low-fat pancakes	1½	2	2½
Maple syrup	½ Tbsp	1 Tbsp	1½ Tbsp

Cottage cheese and cereal

	Under 150 lbs	150–200 lbs	Over 200 lbs
Low-fat cottage cheese	¼ cup	½ cup	¾ cup
Low-fat cereal	6 oz	8 oz	10 oz
Fat-free milk	4 oz	5 oz	6 oz

Cottage cheese and oatmeal

	Under 150 lbs	150–200 lbs	Over 200 lbs
Low-fat cottage cheese	¼ cup	½ cup	¾ cup
Oatmeal	6 oz	8 oz	10 oz
Table sugar	1 Tbsp	1½ Tbsp	2 Tbsp

Carb Refuel Late-Morning Snacks

You should get in more carbs a few hours after your breakfast. Again, stay away from dietary fats because you want to balance the influx of calories you're getting from carbs.

Cereal and treat

	Under 150 lbs	150–200 lbs	Over 200 lbs
Dry cereal	6 oz	8 oz	10 oz
Fat-free milk	4 oz	5 oz	6 oz
Gummi bears	12	15	18

Cottage cheese and an apple

	Under 150 lbs	150–200 lbs	Over 200 lbs
Apple	1 medium	1 medium	1 large
Cottage cheese	¼ cup	½ cup	¾ cup

Protein shake and pretzels

	Under 150 lbs	150–200 lbs	Over 200 lbs
Fat-free pretzels	3 oz	4 oz	5 oz
Whey protein	1 scoop	1½ scoops	2 scoops

Carb Refuel Lunches

For lunch, stay low-fat but include fast-digesting carbs with protein foods. You can add goodies like a soft drink, mashed potatoes, low-fat breads, and any other very low fat to fat-free carbs you can think of, as long as you're getting enough protein with those servings.

Tuna-salad pocket and melon

	Under 150 lbs	150–200 lbs	Over 200 lbs
Light tuna (in water)	½ can	½ can	¾ can
Fat-free mayo	1 Tbsp	1 Tbsp	1 Tbsp
Pita	1 medium	1 large	1 large
Cantaloupe	¼	¼	¼
Regular soda	8 oz	12 oz	16 oz

Chicken with veggies and mashed potatoes

	Under 150 lbs	150–200 lbs	Over 200 lbs
Chicken breast	6 oz	8 oz	10 oz
Mashed potatoes	6 oz	7 oz	8 oz
Steamed veggies	1 cup	1 cup	1 cup

Fish with rice

	Under 150 lbs	150–200 lbs	Over 200 lbs
Cooked whitefish	6 oz	8 oz	10 oz
Cooked brown or white rice	1 cup	1½ cups	2 cups
100% fruit juice (any type)	4 oz	6 oz	8 oz

Turkey with stuffing and sweet potato

	Under 150 lbs	150–200 lbs	Over 200 lbs
Turkey breast	6 oz	8 oz	10 oz
Low-fat stuffing	1 cup	1½ cups	2 cups
Sweet potato	6 oz	7 oz	8 oz

Carb Refuel Midday Snacks

These higher-carb snacks contain virtually no fat. While the options presented are all whole-food meals, they are good choices before workouts. Of course, many people opt to skip the gym on Sundays, but keep in mind that these options can also be selected on workout days during other phases of your nutrition program, because you always want to avoid consuming fats when you're eating your workout meals.

Yogurt

	Under 150 lbs	150–200 lbs	Over 200 lbs
Fat-free yogurt (can contain sugar)	6 oz	8 oz	10 oz

Turkey bagel sandwich

	Under 150 lbs	150–200 lbs	Over 200 lbs
Bagel	1 medium	1 medium	1 large
Low-fat deli turkey meat	3 oz	4 oz	5 oz

Egg and cheese burrito

	Under 150 lbs	150–200 lbs	Over 200 lbs
Egg whites, scrambled	3 large	4 large	5 large
Fat-free cheese	1 oz	1½ oz	2 oz
Fat-free tortilla	1 large	1 large	1 large

Carb Refuel Dinners

Dinners on Carb Refuel days will be lower in fat but much higher in carbs than the dinners during the other nights of the week. While eating carbs later in the day can lead to fat gain, here it will enhance fat loss, as the carbs will help to keep your metabolic rate maximized.

Chicken and pasta with salad

	Under 150 lbs	150–200 lbs	Over 200 lbs
Chicken breast	6 oz	8 oz	10 oz
Cooked spaghetti	¾ cup	1 cup	1¼ cups
Marinara sauce	¼ cup	¼ cup	¼ cup
Green salad	1½ cups	2 cups	2½ cups
Fat-free Italian salad dressing	2 Tbsp	2 Tbsp	2½ Tbsp

Fish with baked potato and peas

	Under 150 lbs	150–200 lbs	Over 200 lbs
Whitefish	6 oz	8 oz	10 oz
Baked potato	1 small	1 medium	1 large
Peas	½ cup	¾ cup	1 cup

Cheeseburger

	Under 150 lbs	150–200 lbs	Over 200 lbs
Extra-lean ground beef	6 oz	8 oz	10 oz
Fat-free American cheese	1 slice	1 slice	1 slice
Hamburger bun	1 medium	1 medium	1 large
Onion	1 slice	1 slice	1 slice
Tomato	1 slice	1 slice	1 slice
Ketchup, mustard, fat-free mayo	To taste	To taste	To taste

Shrimp cocktail, cauliflower, and angel food cake with fruit

	Under 150 lbs	150–200 lbs	Over 200 lbs
Cooked shrimp	6 oz	8 oz	10 oz
Fat-free cocktail sauce	To taste	To taste	To taste
Cauliflower	1 cup	1 cup	1 cup
Individual fat-free angel food cake	½	1	1½
Chopped strawberries	½ cup	½ cup	½ cup
Table sugar	1 Tbsp	1 Tbsp	1 Tbsp

Carb Refuel Nighttime Snacks

Nighttime snacks on your Carb Refuel Sundays differ from the other nighttime snacks because on this day *only* you can eat a moderate amount of carbs before you go to bed. Allow yourself one last treat for the weekend.

Popcorn and cottage cheese

	Under 150 lbs	150–200 lbs	Over 200 lbs
94% fat-free microwave popcorn	¼ bag	⅓ bag	½ bag
Low-fat cottage cheese	¼ cup	½ cup	¾ cup

Deli sandwich

	Under 150 lbs	150–200 lbs	Over 200 lbs
Lean deli meat	3 oz	4 oz	5 oz
White or whole grain bread	1 slice	2 slices	2 slices

Bagel with a smear

	Under 150 lbs	150–200 lbs	Over 200 lbs
Low-fat bagel	1 medium	1 large	1 large
Fat-free cream cheese	3 oz	4 oz	5 oz

CHAPTER 8
MORE PLATINUM 360 RECIPES

In the last chapter, I gave you all sorts of meal options that you can hook up pretty easily, using simple ingredients and prepared foods. The recipes in this section may require a little more effort in the kitchen (not much, I promise), but they offer more varied flavors and have a lot more plate appeal. Each recipe is tagged with one of the five categories listed below, so you can work the dishes into your weekly meal plans.

HEALTHY EATING RECIPES

These can be prepared and eaten on Healthy Eating days of the diet.

Weeks 1 and 2 (and maintenance phase):
Mondays, Tuesdays, and Wednesdays
Weeks 3 and 4: Monday and Tuesday
Weeks 5 and 6: Monday
Weeks 7 and 8: The Healthy Eating phase is not included during these weeks.

Platinum Breakfast Sausage Pizza
Strawberries 'n' Cream Waffle
Scrambled Tofu
Sweet Potato Hash Browns
Crab Boat
Creamy Egg Salad Sandwich
Grown-Up Grilled Cheese
Salmon Pasta Salad
Platinum Power Meatballs 'n' Spaghetti
Chicken Fried Rice
Cheesy Chicken Broccoli Pasta
Taco Salad

TURBOCHARGED FAT BURNING RECIPES

These fit perfectly into your daily meal plan on Turbocharged Fat Burning days of the diet.

Weeks 1 and 2 (and maintenance phase):
Thursdays and Fridays
Weeks 3 and 4: Wednesday, Thursday, and Friday
Weeks 5 and 6: Tuesday, Wednesday, Thursday, and Friday
Weeks 7 and 8: Monday, Tuesday, Wednesday, Thursday, and Friday

If you want to make any of these recipes during your Healthy Eating phase, go ahead and use them as is, or add a small amount of slow-digesting carbs such as oatmeal, fruit, whole grain bread, or brown rice, if you'd like.

Denver Omelet
Feta and Spinach Scramble
LL's Blueberry Protein Pancake
Hearty Breakfast Scramble
Lox Rolls
Broccoli Frittata
Chicken Slaw
Ham 'n' Asparagus Rolls
Mediterranean Tuna Salad
Warm Turkey Wrap
Chopped Chicken Salad
Shrimp Kebabs
Greek-Style Burgers
Spaghetti Squash with Meat Sauce
Salisbury Turkey
Stuffed Peppers
Minced Chicken in Lettuce Cups
Spicy Broiled Salmon

CALORIE RESTRICTION (SATURDAY) RECIPES

All right, you guys, it's the weekend. The recipes in this category can be enjoyed during Calorie Restriction Saturdays. These breakfast and lunch dishes will make the few hours of very low-carb and moderate-fat eating more bearable prior to your Cheat Meal, which follows that evening.

Chicken Fajita Omelet
Spicy Egg White Scramble
Egg and Ham Cup
Tuna in a Cucumber Boat
Shake-No-Bake Shrimp
Spinach Salad with Mustard Vinaigrette

CARB REFUEL (SUNDAY) RECIPES

Keep in mind that all meals you eat on Sundays should not only have plenty of carbs (both fast- and slow-digesting) but also be low in fat (both healthy and saturated).

Platinum Breakfast Sandwich
Savory Buckwheat Pancake
Platinum French Toast
Platinum Turkey Club Sandwich
Platinum Mediterranean Pizza
Chicken Quesadilla
Turkey Chili
Chicken with Egg Noodles
Lemon-Chicken Risotto

ANY-DAY SNACK RECIPES

The snack recipes work any day of the week, regardless of which macronutrient strategy you're following, because they're so low in calories that there aren't enough fats or carbs to keep you from your goal.

Peanut Butter Pudding
Crunchy Cottage Cheese
Crabby Deviled Eggs
Onion Dip
Whole Wheat Tortilla Chips and Cream
  Cheese Dip

BREAKFAST

PLATINUM BREAKFAST SAUSAGE PIZZA

Healthy Eating

Nutrition per serving: Calories: 380 • Protein: 25 g • Carbs: 35 g • Fat: 17 g

Can you think of a better way to start the day than pizza? With a ready-made crust, you can have a delicious and nutritious breakfast in minutes. And you thought this was going to be hard.

¼ Boboli whole wheat pizza crust (12")
1 large egg, lightly beaten
¼ cup shredded reduced-fat mozzarella cheese
2 fully cooked turkey breakfast sausage links (about 2½ ounces each),
    cut into ¼" slices

Preheat the oven to 450°F. Place the crust wedge on a baking sheet. Drizzle half of the egg over the crust, then sprinkle evenly with the cheese. Drizzle the remaining egg over the cheese and arrange the sausage on top. Bake for 10 minutes, or until the cheese is melted and the egg is set.

Makes 1 serving

DENVER OMELET

Turbocharged Fat Burning

Nutrition per serving: Calories: 275 • Protein: 31 g • Carbs: 10 g • Fat: 13 g

This classic breakfast omelet is a great choice during your Turbocharged Fat Burning phase because it is so low in carbs. It's also great at any other time, except when you're trying to avoid fats.

1 teaspoon olive oil
1 large egg
2 large egg whites
¼ onion, diced
½ green bell pepper, diced
3 ounces cooked ham, diced

In a medium nonstick skillet, heat the oil over medium-high heat. In a small bowl, beat the whole egg and egg whites until well combined. Add the eggs to the pan and cook, without stirring, until set on the bottom. Sprinkle with the onion, pepper, and ham, then slide a spatula underneath and fold the omelet in half. Cook until the eggs are completely set.

Makes 1 serving

STRAWBERRIES 'N' CREAM WAFFLE

Nutrition per serving: Calories: 171 • Protein: 4 g • Carbs: 33 g • Fat: 3 g

This breakfast is so good you'll feel like you're cheating, but the slow-digesting carbs in this whole grain and fruit treat won't end up on your hips or belly. If you're really slick, you can make the waffle from a whole grain mix. Since this item is mainly a carbohydrate, serve with scrambled eggs or one of the Turbocharged Fat Burning or Calorie Restriction (Saturday) recipes to make it a complete breakfast.

1 frozen whole grain waffle

1 cup sliced strawberries

1 tablespoon 0% plain Greek yogurt

1 teaspoon light brown sugar

Toast the waffle as directed and top with the strawberries. In a small bowl, stir together the yogurt and brown sugar and dollop on top of the waffle.

Makes 1 serving

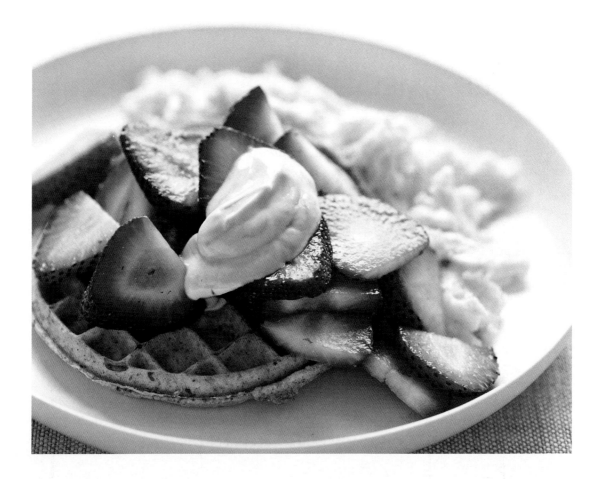

SCRAMBLED TOFU

Nutrition per serving: Calories: 313 • Protein: 22 g • Carbs: 26 g • Fat: 15 g

I know what you're thinking: Tofu? But silken tofu has a custardlike texture, and it scrambles up into a tasty egg substitute. The curry adds potent antioxidants that boost health and recovery.

1 teaspoon olive oil

2 scallions, sliced

1 green bell pepper, diced

½ red bell pepper, diced

1 teaspoon reduced-sodium soy sauce

½ teaspoon curry powder

1 package (12.3 ounces) silken tofu, drained and mashed lightly
   with a fork

2 tablespoons 2% plain Greek yogurt

2 tablespoons tomato salsa

In a large nonstick skillet, heat the oil over medium heat. Add half of the scallions and cook, stirring often, until translucent, about 1 minute. Add the peppers, soy sauce, curry powder, and tofu and cook, stirring, until hot. Serve topped with the yogurt, salsa, and remaining scallions.

Makes 1 serving

SWEET POTATO HASH BROWNS

Nutrition per serving: Calories: 171• Protein: 3 g• Carbs: 30 g• Fat: 5 g

White potatoes are nutritional wastelands, but their orange brethren are packed with nutrients—notably, beta-carotene—and are slow-digesting to boot. That means sweet potatoes can be included in many Healthy Eating recipes. Since this item is mainly a carbohydrate, serve it with eggs, such as scrambled eggs or one of the Turbocharged Fat Burning or Calorie Restriction (Saturday) breakfast recipes, to make it a complete breakfast.

   1 sweet potato (about 7 ounces), peeled and shredded
¼ onion, shredded
½ green bell pepper, finely chopped
Salt and ground black pepper
1 teaspoon olive oil

In a medium bowl, stir together the sweet potato, onion, and bell pepper. Season with salt and black pepper to taste.

In a large nonstick skillet, heat the oil over medium-high heat. Add the sweet potato mixture and cook, stirring occasionally, until the potatoes are lightly browned.

Makes 1 serving

FETA AND SPINACH SCRAMBLE

Nutrition per serving: Calories: 225 • Protein: 29 g • Carbs: 3 g • Fat: 10 g

Ever been to the Mediterranean? No need to book tickets—just zip up your breakfast with this feta and spinach scrambled egg dish and you'll feel like you just landed.

   1 tablespoon olive oil
1 large egg
2 large egg whites
2 ounces reduced-fat feta cheese
1 cup chopped fresh spinach
1 slow-digesting carb source (optional): 1 slice whole wheat or Ezekiel 4:9
     toast, a piece of fruit, or oatmeal

In a medium skillet, heat the oil over medium-high heat. In a small bowl, whisk the whole egg and egg whites until well combined. Add the eggs to the pan and gently scramble as they begin to set. Add the cheese and spinach and cook to your preferred doneness.

Makes 1 serving

LL'S BLUEBERRY PROTEIN PANCAKE

Turbocharged Fat Burning

Nutrition per serving: Calories: 167 • Protein: 32 g • Carbs: 10 g • Fat: 0 g

Get ready to satisfy your early morning sweet tooth with this delicious low-carb pancake. You'll also add high-quality muscle-building protein to your diet.

1 scoop (31 g) vanilla whey protein

1 tablespoon 1% milk

3 large egg whites

½ teaspoon ground cinnamon

¼ teaspoon salt

½ teaspoon baking powder

¼ cup blueberries

1 tablespoon sugar-free pancake syrup

In a medium bowl, combine the whey protein, milk, egg whites, cinnamon, salt, and baking powder, whisking to combine. Add the blueberries and then set the batter aside for 2 minutes.

Coat a small nonstick skillet with cooking spray and heat over medium heat. Pour all of the batter into the skillet to make 1 large pancake and cook until lightly browned on both sides, 1 to 2 minutes per side. Serve topped with the pancake syrup.

Makes 1 serving

HEARTY BREAKFAST SCRAMBLE

Nutrition per serving: Calories: 300 • Protein: 34 g • Carbs: 5 g • Fat: 12 g

Get your morning started right with protein-packed eggs and lean meat (be sure to include a slow-digesting carb source, such as 1 slice of whole wheat or Ezekiel 4:9 toast, a piece of fruit, or oatmeal). The Parmesan cheese adds a salty bite that'll get you ready for the day. You'll have to find your car keys on your own, though.

¼ pound lean ground beef or turkey breast

¼ onion, chopped

1 large egg, lightly beaten

¼ cup grated Parmesan cheese

2 tablespoons fat-free sour cream

In a large nonstick skillet, cook the ground meat and onion over medium heat, stirring occasionally, until completely browned, 3 to 4 minutes. Stir in the egg and cook for about 1 minute, then stir in the cheese. Transfer to a plate and serve topped with the sour cream.

Makes 1 serving

LOX ROLLS

Nutrition per serving: Calories: 232 • Protein: 29 g • Carbs: 1 g • Fat: 11 g

Guaranteed your coffee has never met bagels like these. At least you can think of them as bagels, just without the carbs (and with a lot of protein).

1 large egg

2 large egg whites

2 tablespoons chopped fresh chives

2 slices (2 ounces total) lox (smoked salmon)

In a small bowl, beat the whole egg, egg whites, and chives until well combined.

Coat a medium nonstick skillet with cooking spray and heat over medium heat. Pour the egg mixture into the pan and scramble to your preferred doneness. Spoon some of the eggs over each lox slice and roll like a cigar. Serve while the eggs are hot.

Makes 1 serving

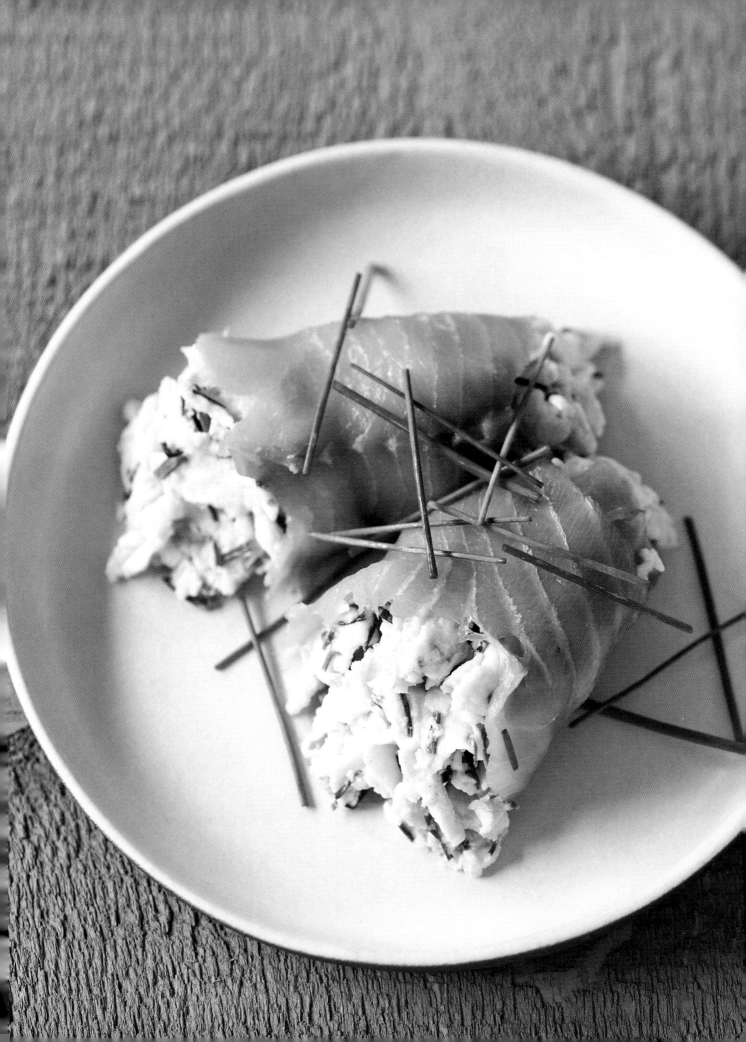

BROCCOLI FRITTATA

Nutrition per serving: Calories: 336 • Protein: 28 g • Carbs: 12 g • Fat: 20 g

Craving veggies in the morning? Add some to your breakfast with this easy-to-make egg dish that's low in carbs. Serve it with a slow-digesting carb source, such as 1 slice of whole wheat or Ezekiel 4:9 toast, a piece of fruit, or oatmeal.

1 tablespoon olive oil
½ onion, chopped
1 cup chopped fresh broccoli
1 large egg
1 large egg white
½ cup 2% cottage cheese

In a large skillet, heat the oil over medium heat. Add the onion and broccoli and cook until the vegetables are softened, about 5 minutes.

Meanwhile, in a bowl, whisk the whole egg and egg white together until well combined. Stir in the cottage cheese.

Add the egg mixture to the skillet, then lift and rotate the pan so that the eggs are evenly distributed. As the eggs begin to set, use a spatula to lift the edges to allow uncooked egg to run underneath. Turn the heat to low, cover the pan, and cook until the top is set, 3 to 5 minutes. Invert the frittata onto a plate.

Makes 1 serving

CHICKEN FAJITA OMELET

Nutrition per serving: Calories: 225 • Protein: 33 g • Carbs: 8 g • Fat: 5 g

Remember Saturday morning cartoons? Now you have something to look forward to on Saturday mornings again. Spice up your breakfast with this fajita-inspired omelet.

1 large egg
1 large egg white
2 ounces cooked chicken
½ cup shredded fat-free Cheddar cheese
¼ red bell pepper, cut into thin strips
¼ onion, thinly sliced

¼ teaspoon chili powder

2 tablespoons salsa

1 tablespoon fat-free sour cream

Coat a medium nonstick skillet with cooking spray and heat over medium heat. In a small bowl, whisk the whole egg and egg white until fluffy. Add the eggs to the pan and cook without stirring until set on the bottom.

Flip the omelet and top with the chicken, cheese, pepper, onion, and chili powder. Fold the omelet over the filling and cook for 1 to 2 minutes. Flip again and cook until the cheese is melted and the filling is heated through, 1 to 2 minutes. Slide the omelet onto a plate and top with the salsa and sour cream.

Makes 1 serving

SPICY EGG WHITE SCRAMBLE

Nutrition per serving: Calories: 152 • Protein: 28 g • Carbs: 2 g • Fat: 3 g

Mixing egg whites with spicy salsa not only helps rev up your metabolism but makes low-calorie egg whites seem more satisfying. And that added energy boost will come in handy, because that lawn ain't cutting itself.

6 large egg whites

¼ cup spicy salsa

¼ cup shredded reduced-fat mozzarella cheese

Coat a large nonstick skillet with cooking spray and heat over medium heat. In a medium bowl, beat the egg whites until well combined. Stir in the salsa and cheese and mix well. Add the egg mixture to the pan and scramble to your preferred degree of doneness.

Makes 1 serving

EGG AND HAM CUP

Nutrition per serving: Calories: 164 • Protein: 24 g • Carbs: 2 g • Fat: 6 g

Easy-to-make Saturday morning treats—because seriously, who wants to work hard in the kitchen after the week you just had?

1 slice 97% fat-free deli-sliced ham
1 slice tomato
1 large egg
1 large egg white
¼ cup shredded fat-free Cheddar cheese

Preheat the oven to 375°F. Spray 1 cup of a muffin tin with cooking spray. Press the ham slice into the muffin tin, forming a cup. Place the tomato slice in the cup, then crack the whole egg and drop it in on top of the tomato. Crack the second egg, letting just the egg white fall into the cup (discard the yolk).

Bake the ham cup for 10 to 15 minutes, or until the egg is almost cooked. Top with the cheese and bake for 3 to 5 minutes to melt the cheese. Let cool for a few minutes, then use a spatula to transfer carefully to a plate.

Makes 1 serving

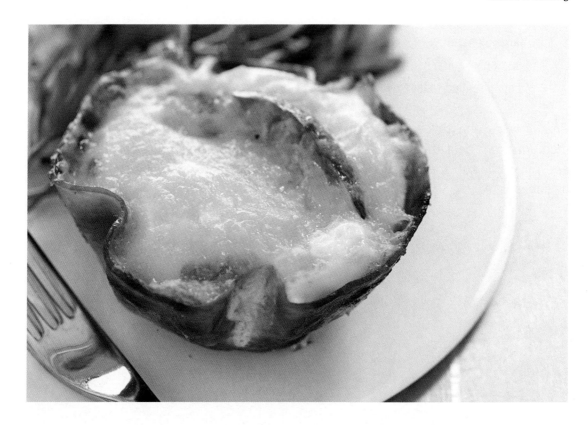

PLATINUM BREAKFAST SANDWICH

Nutrition per serving: Calories: 304 • Protein: 30 g • Carbs: 33 g • Fat: 5 g

This breakfast sandwich tastes even better than a fast-food egg-on-a-muffin, and it won't blow up your waistband or your heart (though it could find a place there).

    2 slices extra-lean turkey bacon
    1 large egg
    1 slice (⅔ ounce) reduced-fat cheese
    1 English muffin, toasted
    1 slice tomato

Coat a small nonstick skillet with cooking spray. Add the turkey bacon and cook until crisp, about 7 minutes.

Coat a second small nonstick skillet with cooking spray and place over medium heat. Break the egg into the skillet and cook until nearly set, then top with the cheese and cook until the egg is done to your liking and the cheese is warm.

Place the cheese-topped egg on 1 half of the English muffin top with the turkey bacon, tomato, and the other English muffin half.

Makes 1 serving

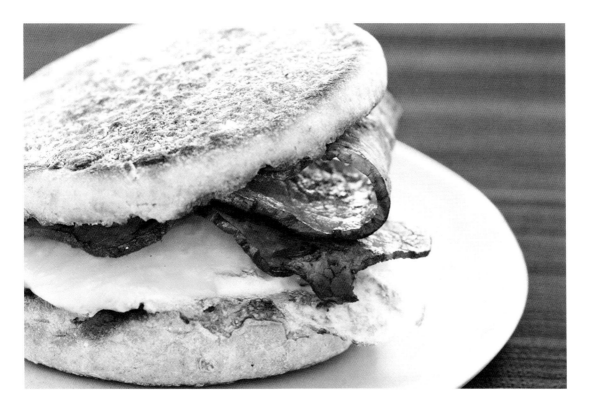

SAVORY BUCKWHEAT PANCAKE

Nutrition per serving: Calories: 420 • Protein: 30 g • Carbs: 32 g • Fat: 5 g

Buckwheat flour gives this pancake extra protein power as well as nutrients that knock out fat and can help lower cholesterol levels. You'll feel yourself getting healthy.

⅓ cup buckwheat pancake mix (such as Aunt Jemima)

1 large egg white

1 cup 1% milk

1 tablespoon vegetable oil

2 large eggs

3 slices extra-lean turkey bacon

¼ cup shredded fat-free cheese

Maple syrup (optional)

In a large bowl, prepare the pancake batter according to package directions, using the egg white and the milk.

In a small bowl, whisk the eggs until blended. Coat a medium nonstick skillet with cooking spray and place over medium heat. Add the eggs and scramble until cooked to your liking.

Coat a small nonstick skillet with cooking spray and heat over medium heat. Cook the turkey bacon until crisp, 5 to 7 minutes.

Coat a large nonstick skillet with cooking spray and heat over medium-high heat. Pour all of the pancake batter into the pan to form 1 large pancake. Cook until the bottom is browned, about 2 minutes, then flip the pancake and top with the scrambled eggs, bacon, and cheese. Cook until the bottom of the pancake is browned and cooked, fold the pancake in half over the filling, and serve. Top with maple syrup, if desired.

Makes 1 serving

PLATINUM FRENCH TOAST

Nutrition per serving: Calories: 353• Protein: 24 g• Carbs: 46 g• Fat: 8 g

On Sundays you can treat yourself to this high-carb special—while it's packed with protein, it's also low in fat. Your sweet tooth will thank you for the punch of cinnamon, too.

1 large egg

2 large egg whites

¼ cup 1% milk

½ teaspoon ground cinnamon

½ teaspoon vanilla extract

2 slices (1 ounce each) whole wheat bread

1 tablespoon confectioners' sugar or maple syrup

¼ cup fresh berries

In a shallow bowl, whisk together the whole egg and egg whites until well combined. Whisk in the milk, cinnamon, and vanilla extract.

Coat a medium nonstick skillet with cooking spray and place over medium-high heat. Dunk the bread slices into the egg mixture, add to the skillet, and cook until golden, about 1½ minutes per side.

Serve topped with the confectioners' sugar and berries.

Makes 1 serving

LUNCH

Healthy Eating

CRAB BOAT

Nutrition per serving: Calories: 300 • Protein: 26 g • Carbs: 35 g • Fat: 7 g

Love crabs? Pop one of these babies and you'll think you're sitting on the Eastern Shore of the Chesapeake.

    4 ounces lump crabmeat, picked over to remove cartilage
    1 celery rib, chopped
    ¼ onion, chopped
    1 tablespoon light mayonnaise
    1 teaspoon fresh lemon juice
    1 whole wheat pita (6")
    1 romaine or iceberg lettuce leaf

In a large bowl, combine the crabmeat, celery, onion, mayonnaise, and lemon juice and mix well. Carefully slice open the top of the pita. Place the lettuce inside and stuff with the crab mixture.

Makes 1 serving

Healthy Eating

CREAMY EGG SALAD SANDWICH

Nutrition per serving: Calories: 300 • Protein: 28 g • Carbs: 30 g • Fat: 9 g

This egg salad is so rich and creamy it will seem like you're eating a decadent sandwich, but you're actually fueling your body with quality protein and slow-digesting carbs.

    2 large eggs, hard-boiled
    ¼ cup 2% cottage cheese
    ¼ cup 2% plain Greek yogurt
    1 tablespoon Dijon mustard
    2 slices (1 ounce each) whole wheat bread, toasted
    4 thin slices cucumber

Halve the eggs and discard one of the yolks. Place the egg whites and yolk in a medium bowl and mash with a fork. Add the cottage cheese, yogurt, and mustard and mix thoroughly. Make a sandwich with the bread, cucumber, and egg mixture.

Makes 1 serving

GROWN-UP GRILLED CHEESE

Nutrition per serving: Calories: 415• Protein: 45 g• Carbs: 43 g• Fat: 7 g

Now I'm gonna bring you back to your childhood. Come on, who didn't love Mom's grilled cheese? But this one is packed with protein, so your muscles will love you. Oh, it's delicious, too. Just like your mama's.

- 1 tablespoon Dijon mustard
- 2 slices (1 ounce each) whole wheat bread
- ¼ pound deli-sliced chicken breast
- 2 slices (1 ounce each) reduced-fat Swiss cheese
- 1 cup low-sodium tomato soup

Spread the mustard on both slices of bread. Top the bread in this order: 1 slice of the cheese, all of the chicken, and the second slice of cheese.

Coat a medium skillet with cooking spray and heat over medium heat. Place the sandwich in the skillet and cook until golden brown, 2 to 3 minutes per side. Serve with the tomato soup.

Makes 1 serving

CHICKEN SLAW

Nutrition per serving: Calories: 255 • Protein: 30 g • Carbs: 8 g • Fat: 12 g

Time to do that boring old coleslaw some favors. This recipe gives an extra dose of protein to coleslaw and turns this side dish into a meal. On moderate- or high-carb days, serve as a sandwich on 2 slices of whole wheat or Ezekiel 4:9 bread.

- 1 tablespoon light mayonnaise
- 1 tablespoon apple cider vinegar
- Salt and ground black pepper
- 6 ounces cooked chicken breast, diced or shredded
- 1 cup coleslaw mix

In a medium bowl, whisk together the mayonnaise and vinegar. Season with salt and pepper to taste. Add the chicken and coleslaw mix and toss well.

Makes 1 serving

SALMON PASTA SALAD

Nutrition per serving: Calories: 450• Protein: 29 g• Carbs: 44 g• Fat: 16 g

Here we take pasta and kick it up a notch by dropping in some salmon to provide pro-tein and essential fats, two must-have nutrients for muscle recovery and health. Unlike its refined-flour counterparts, whole grain pasta provides a slow, steady release of energy.

3 ounces salmon fillet, skinless

2 ounces whole wheat elbow macaroni

¼ cup frozen peas, thawed

¼ onion, chopped

½ tomato, chopped

1 tablespoon light mayonnaise

Preheat the broiler. Line a broiler pan with foil. Broil the salmon for 5 to 7 minutes, or until it is just barely cooked through. Set aside to cool.

Bring a large pot of water to a boil. Add the macaroni and cook according to package direc-tions. Drain and rinse under cold running water; drain well. Transfer to a large bowl.

Add the reserved salmon, peas, onion, tomato, and mayonnaise to the pasta and mix thor-oughly, making sure the salmon has flaked apart into small pieces and is well distributed. Serve at room temperature or refrigerate to chill.

Makes 1 serving

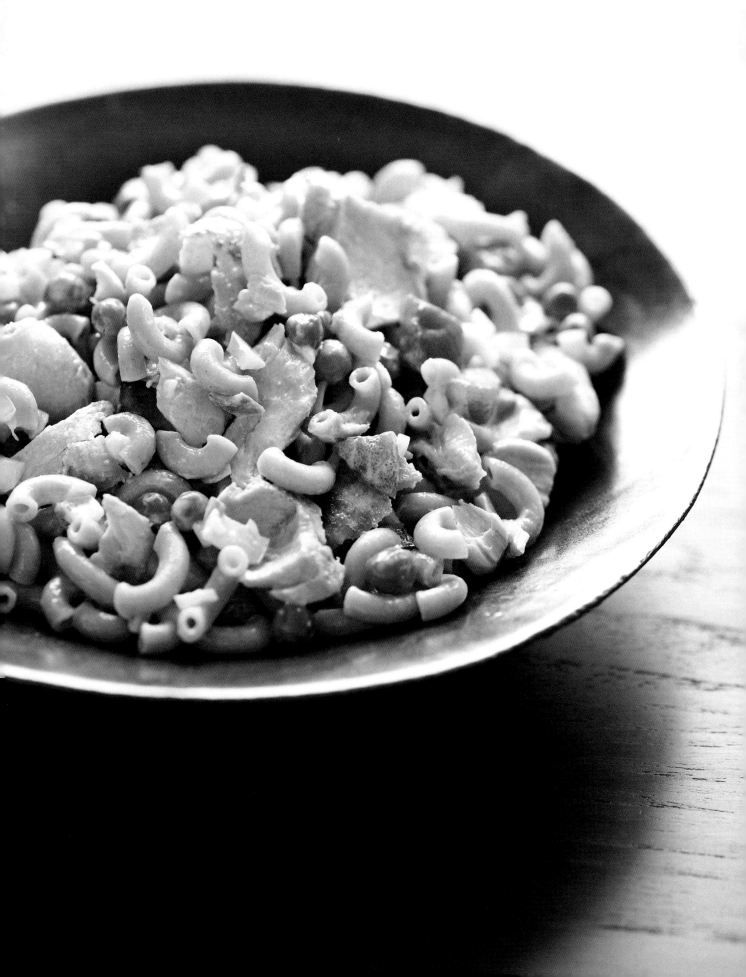

HAM 'N' ASPARAGUS ROLLS

Nutrition per serving: Calories: 237 • Protein: 34 g • Carbs: 10 g • Fat: 6 g

You can go all out and use fresh steamed asparagus—or go the canned asparagus route to make this a no-cook dish. Either way, the rolls are fun to make. And who says good health isn't fun?

 3 fresh asparagus spears
 3 slices (1 ounce each) 97% fat-free deli ham or turkey breast
 3 slices (1 ounce each) reduced-fat cheese
 1½ tablespoons fat-free cream cheese

Bring ½" of water to a boil in a steamer or skillet. Add the asparagus and steam until crisp-tender, 1 to 2 minutes. Remove and set aside to cool.

Place 1 slice of the ham on a plate or cutting board. Lay 1 slice of the cheese on top and spread with 1½ teaspoons of the cream cheese. Place an asparagus spear along 1 edge and roll the ham and cheese around the asparagus. Repeat with the remaining ingredients.

Makes 1 serving

MEDITERRANEAN TUNA SALAD

Nutrition per serving: Calories: 165 • Protein: 28 g • Carbs: 7 g • Fat: 2 g

Unlike the fatty tuna salad you get at most restaurants, this version swaps out mayo for lemon juice and adds some healthy fats from olives—an easy fix that goes a long way toward eating better. On moderate- or high-carb days, serve the tuna salad as a sandwich on 2 slices of whole wheat or Ezekiel 4:9 bread.

 1 can (5 ounces) water-packed chunk light tuna, drained
 ½ tomato, chopped
 ½ cup chopped cucumber
 2 tablespoons chopped red onion
 4 large pitted black olives, chopped
 3 tablespoons fresh lemon juice
 Salt and ground black pepper
 Mixed salad greens

Place the tuna in a bowl and break it up with a fork. Add the tomato, cucumber, onion, olives, and lemon juice. Season with salt and pepper to taste and mix thoroughly. Serve over a bed of mixed greens.

Makes 2 servings

WARM TURKEY WRAP

Turbocharged
Fat Burning

Nutrition per serving: Calories: 300 • Protein: 34 g • Carbs*: 18 g • Fat: 8 g

This wrap will not only warm you up on cold days but will make your low-carb days feel like you haven't made any sacrifices in your carb intake. And it might even warm your heart.

  1 low-carb tortilla (8")
  1 tablespoon light mayonnaise
  ¼ pound deli-sliced turkey breast
  1 slice (1 ounce) reduced-fat Swiss cheese
  1 romaine lettuce leaf
  3 sweet cherry peppers, sliced

Warm the tortilla in a dry skillet, turning until it is pliable and starting to blister. Remove the tortilla from the skillet and quickly spread with the mayonnaise. Top with the turkey, cheese, lettuce, and peppers. Roll the tortilla around the filling and eat warm.

Makes 1 serving

*The low-carb tortilla provides 12 of the 18 grams of total carbs here, but 8 of those grams are from fiber, which means that you are really only consuming 10 grams of net carbs.

CHOPPED CHICKEN SALAD

Nutrition per serving: Calories: 436 • Protein: 30 g • Carbs: 12 g • Fat: 30 g

This salad provides good protein and fats to keep you energized on lower-carb days. You didn't think I'd let you sacrifice your energy now, did you?

2 cups mixed greens

½ tomato, chopped

¼ red onion, chopped

2 ounces cooked chicken breast, chopped

1 hard-boiled egg, peeled and chopped

2 slices extra-lean turkey bacon, cooked and chopped

¼ Hass avocado, sliced

2 tablespoons olive oil

Balsamic vinegar

In a large bowl, combine the greens, tomato, and onion. Top with the chicken, egg, bacon, and avocado. Drizzle with the oil and vinegar to taste and toss well.

Makes 1 serving

TUNA IN A CUCUMBER BOAT

Nutrition per serving: Calories: 165 • Protein: 29 g • Carbs: 8 g • Fat: 1 g

When you're going low-calorie, crunchy low-carb vegetables can really keep those carb cravings in check. Cucumbers make a great cracker or bread substitute.

1 can (5 ounces) water-packed chunk light tuna, drained

2 tablespoons chopped red onion

2 tablespoons shredded carrot

1 tablespoon fat-free plain yogurt

1 tablespoon fresh lemon juice

Salt and ground black pepper

½ cucumber, halved lengthwise and seeded

In a small bowl, stir together the tuna, onion, carrot, yogurt, and lemon juice. Season with salt and pepper to taste. Mix to combine.

Divide the tuna mixture between the cucumber halves, spooning it down the middle.

Makes 1 serving

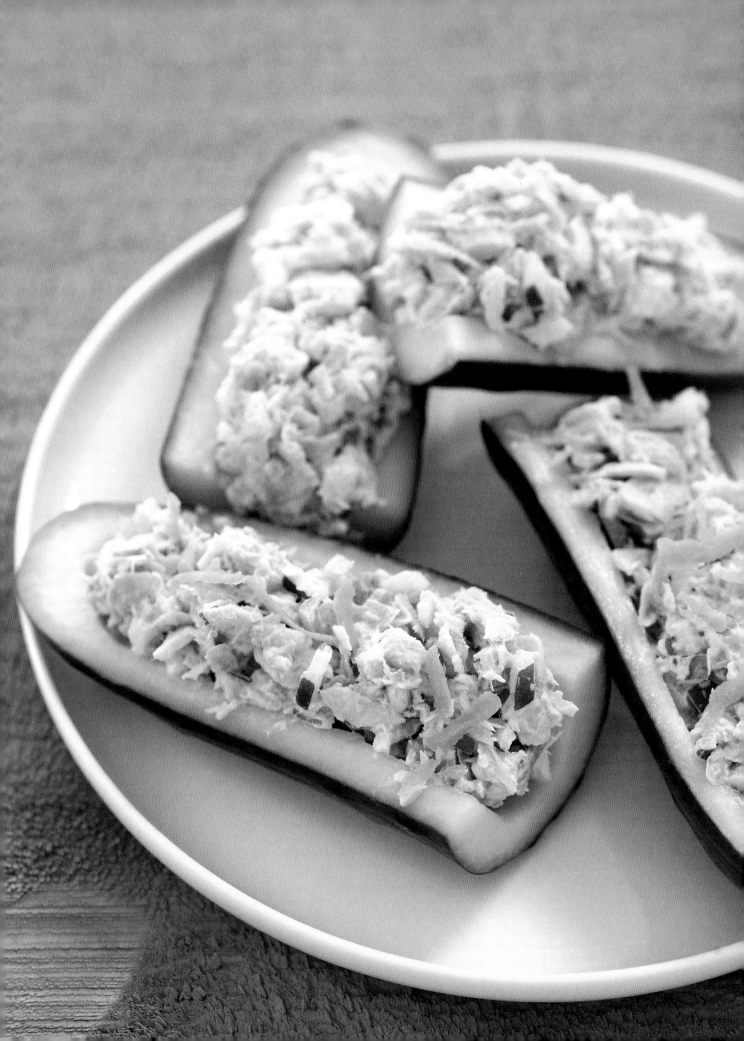

SHAKE-NO-BAKE SHRIMP

Nutrition per serving: Calories: 180 • Protein: 35 g • Carbs: 1 g • Fat: 3 g

This easy-to-make shrimp recipe is so good it will feel like you're spoiling yourself, so you'll never miss the carbs. Come on, you deserve it.

6 ounces cooked peeled shrimp

½ teaspoon garlic powder

½ teaspoon onion powder

½ teaspoon grated lemon zest

Salt and ground black pepper

Place the shrimp, garlic powder, onion powder, lemon zest, and salt and pepper to taste in a quart-size resealable plastic bag. Shake the bag to coat the shrimp with the seasonings. Marinate for 15 minutes in the refrigerator before serving.

Makes 1 serving

SPINACH SALAD WITH MUSTARD VINAIGRETTE

Nutrition per serving: Calories: 208 • Protein: 28 g • Carbs*: 12 g • Fat: 2.5 g

This salad is the perfect lunch for this restrictive day, not to mention that it's easy to put together. Keeping it simple—and tasty.

2 tablespoons apple cider vinegar

1 tablespoon Dijon mustard

1 tablespoon fat-free plain yogurt

Salt and ground black pepper

3 ounces cooked chicken breast, shredded or chopped

10 asparagus spears, steamed and chopped

½ cucumber, diced

¼ red onion, thinly sliced

2 cups baby spinach

In a medium bowl, whisk together the vinegar, mustard, and yogurt. Season with salt and pepper to taste. Add the chicken, asparagus, cucumber, onion, and spinach. Toss to combine.

Makes 1 serving

*Although this meal provides 12 grams of total carbs, 7 of those grams come from fiber, which means that you are really consuming only 5 grams of net carbs.

PLATINUM TURKEY CLUB SANDWICH

Carb Refuel
Sunday

Nutrition per serving: Calories: 400 • Protein: 43 g • Carbs: 42 g • Fat: 7 g

Bet you thought club sandwiches were off-limits on low-fat days. Would I do that to you? This double-decker stacks up the protein and carbs to satisfy the biggest appetite.

   3 slices (1 ounce each) whole wheat bread
   1 tablespoon mustard
   4 slices deli turkey breast
   4 slices extra-lean turkey bacon, cooked
   ½ tomato, sliced
   1 cup shredded iceberg lettuce

Place 1 slice of bread on a plate and spread with 1½ teaspoons of the mustard. Top with 2 slices of the turkey, 2 slices of the bacon, half of the tomato slices, and ½ cup of the lettuce. Place a second slice of bread on top and spread with the remaining 1½ teaspoons mustard. Stack the remaining turkey, bacon, tomato, and lettuce on top and finish with the third slice of bread. Cut the sandwich in half on the diagonal.

Makes 1 serving

PLATINUM MEDITERRANEAN PIZZA

Nutrition per serving: Calories: 404 • Protein: 34 g • Carbs: 48 g • Fat: 9 g

I see you trying to hide those Pizza Hut coupons. Toss 'em. Because this high-protein homemade pie gives you plenty of carbs with little fat. Cut your arteries a huge break, my friend.

¼ Boboli whole wheat pizza crust (12")
¼ cup marinara sauce
¼ cup fat-free ricotta cheese
2 ounces cooked chicken sausage, thinly sliced
¼ onion, thinly sliced
4 large pitted black olives, sliced
Pinch of dried oregano

Preheat the oven to 450°F. Place the pizza crust on a baking sheet. Spread the marinara evenly over the crust. Top with dollops of ricotta, the chicken sausage, onion, and olives. Sprinkle with the oregano and bake for 10 to 15 minutes, or until the crust is crisp.

Makes 1 serving

CHICKEN QUESADILLA

Nutrition per serving: Calories: 320 • Protein: 33 g • Carbs: 33 g • Fat: 5 g

Time to enjoy some banging Mexican fare with this healthy quesadilla—low in fat, with flavor off the charts.

1 large whole wheat tortilla (10")
2 ounces cooked chicken breast, chopped
¼ cup shredded fat-free Monterey Jack cheese
1 poblano chile pepper, sliced
¼ cup salsa

Heat a large skillet over medium heat and add the tortilla. Cover 1 side of the tortilla with the chicken, cheese, and pepper. Fold the tortilla in half over the filling. Cook for 2 to 3 minutes on 1 side, then turn and cook on the other side until the cheese is melted. Serve topped with the salsa.

Makes 1 serving

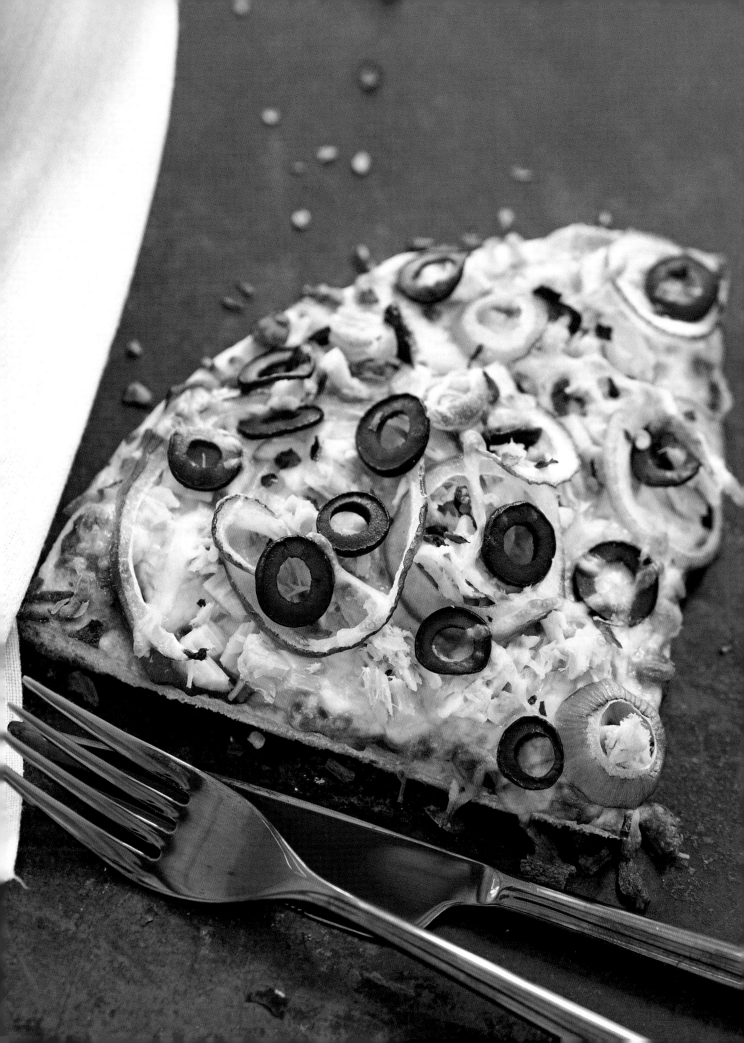

DINNER

PLATINUM POWER MEATBALLS 'N' SPAGHETTI

Nutrition per serving: Calories: 383 • Protein: 35 g • Carbs: 38 g • Fat: 9 g

By substituting wheat germ for some bread crumbs, these meatballs will bring the power. Wheat germ is a very slow-digesting carb that also contains a natural plant ingredient called octacosanol. Translation: increased muscle strength and endurance. That's a good thing.

1 pound extra-lean ground beef or turkey breast

1 large egg

¼ cup plain wheat germ

¼ cup Italian-style bread crumbs

Salt and ground black pepper

1 jar (26 ounces) marinara sauce

8 ounces whole wheat spaghetti

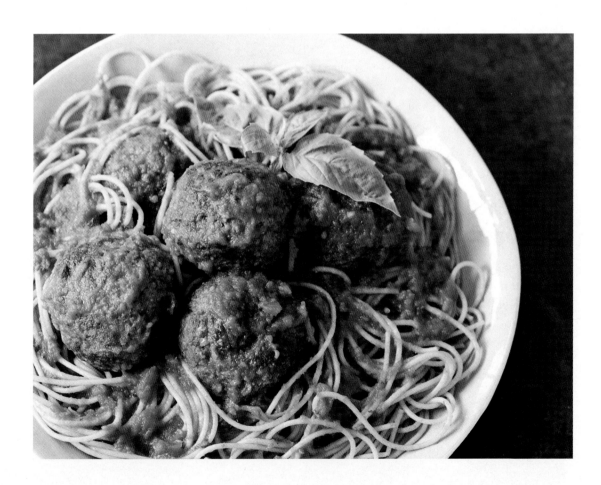

In a large bowl, combine the beef, egg, wheat germ, and bread crumbs. Season with salt and pepper to taste. Mix gently until combined. Form into 16 small (or 8 large) meatballs.

Coat a large nonstick skillet with cooking spray and heat over medium-high heat. Add the meatballs and turn to brown all sides. Add the marinara to the pan, reduce the heat to a simmer, cover, and cook, stirring occasionally, until the meatballs are cooked through, 15 to 20 minutes.

Meanwhile, bring a large pot of water to a boil. Add the pasta and cook according to package directions. Drain the pasta and serve topped with the meatballs and sauce.

Makes 4 servings

CHICKEN FRIED RICE

Nutrition per serving: Calories: 416 • Protein: 38 g • Carbs: 35 g • Fat: 12 g

You could make this dish from scratch, but using it to bring new life to leftover brown rice and cooked chicken saves you time in the kitchen.

1 teaspoon olive oil
1 large egg, beaten
¼ onion, chopped
½ cup frozen peas and carrots
4 ounces cooked chicken breast, cubed
½ cup cooked brown rice
2 tablespoons reduced-sodium soy sauce

In a large nonstick skillet, heat the oil over medium heat. Add the egg and gently scramble. Transfer the egg to a plate.

Add the onion and vegetables to the same skillet and cook until the onion is translucent, 3 to 5 minutes. Add the chicken, rice, and soy sauce. Continue to cook and stir until the ingredients are warmed through. Return the egg to the skillet and toss to mix.

Makes 1 serving

CHEESY CHICKEN BROCCOLI PASTA

Nutrition per serving: Calories: 393 • Protein: 45 g • Carbs: 35 g • Fat: 8 g

Don't be afraid of broccoli. We're going to sprinkle it in with some protein-packed chicken for a delicious way to do pasta.

> 1 cup whole wheat penne
> 1 teaspoon olive oil
> ¼ medium onion, sliced
> ¼ pound boneless, skinless chicken breast, cubed
> 1 cup broccoli florets
> ½ cup part-skim ricotta cheese

Bring a large saucepan of water to a boil. Add the pasta and cook according to package directions. Reserving ¼ cup of the cooking water, drain the pasta.

In a large nonstick skillet, heat the oil over medium-high heat. Add the onion and chicken and cook until the chicken is cooked through, about 5 minutes.

Meanwhile, in a steamer, cook the broccoli until crisp-tender, about 2 minutes.

In a medium bowl, whisk the reserved pasta cooking water into the ricotta until smooth. Add the pasta, chicken, and broccoli and toss to coat.

Makes 1 serving

SHRIMP KEBABS

Nutrition per serving: Calories: 365 • Protein: 38 g • Carbs: 16 g • Fat: 17 g

These zesty shrimp kebabs will have you looking forward to low-carb dinners. These things are so good you'll flip. Just put the skewers down first.

> ¼ cup olive oil
> ¼ cup reduced-sodium soy sauce
> ¼ cup fresh lemon juice
> 1 teaspoon garlic powder
> 6 ounces peeled and deveined shrimp
> ½ onion, cut into 1" chunks and separated into pieces
> ½ zucchini, cut into ½" pieces

In a large bowl, stir together the oil, soy sauce, lemon juice, and garlic powder. Add the shrimp, stir to coat with the marinade, and refrigerate for 30 minutes to 1 hour.

Preheat a stovetop grill pan or an outdoor grill until very hot. Thread the shrimp onto skewers, alternating them with the onion and zucchini chunks. Grill the skewers just until the shrimp turn pink, about 2 minutes per side.

Makes 1 serving

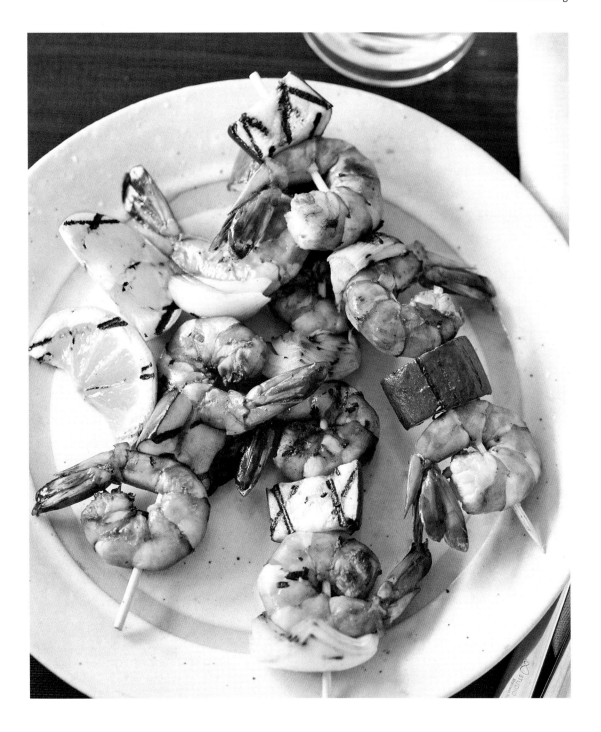

TACO SALAD

Nutrition per serving: Calories: 343 • Protein: 36 g • Carbs: 30 g • Fat: 11 g

Sure, you could roll up the ingredients in a tortilla, but eating it open-faced with a fork and knife lets you pile on more vegetables. That means more vitamins and healthy fiber, which will keep you fuller for longer.

   1 whole wheat tortilla (8")
   ¼ onion, diced
   ¼ pound lean ground beef
   2 teaspoons chili powder
   Salt and ground black pepper
   2 tablespoons shredded reduced-fat Cheddar cheese
   2 cups chopped romaine lettuce
   ½ green bell pepper, sliced
   ½ red bell pepper, sliced
   1 tablespoon low-fat ranch dressing
   2 tablespoons tomato salsa

If desired, toast the tortilla in a toaster oven or dry skillet until browned and crispy.

Coat a large skillet with cooking spray and heat over medium-high heat. Add the onion, beef, chili powder, and salt and pepper to taste. Cook, breaking up the meat with a spoon, until browned, 3 to 5 minutes.

To serve, place the tortilla on a plate and top with the beef mixture, cheese, lettuce, and bell peppers. Top with the ranch dressing and salsa.

Makes 1 serving

GREEK-STYLE BURGERS

Nutrition per serving: Calories: 284 • Protein: 35 g • Carbs: 7 g • Fat: 13 g

This recipe will put your boring burgers to shame. These bad boys bring the flavors of the Greek isles to your table. Serve with vegetables and/or a mixed green salad.

   1 pound lean ground beef or turkey
   2 cups chopped spinach
   ½ cup Italian-style bread crumbs
   ½ cup fat-free feta cheese

1 large egg

1 tablespoon tomato paste

Salt and ground black pepper

Preheat the grill or broiler.

In a large bowl, combine the ground meat, spinach, bread crumbs, cheese, egg, tomato paste, and salt and pepper to taste. Mix gently but thoroughly. Shape into 4 burgers and grill or broil for 4 to 5 minutes per side, or until cooked through.

Makes 4 servings

SPAGHETTI SQUASH WITH MEAT SAUCE

Turbocharged Fat Burning

Nutrition per serving: Calories: 320 • Protein: 27 g • Carbs: 16 g • Fat: 19 g

With a hearty meat sauce on top, you might find that you actually prefer the crisp, fresh flavor of spaghetti squash to pasta. No need to thank me for broadening your horizons.

1 small spaghetti squash (about 2 pounds)

1 teaspoon olive oil

¼ onion, diced

2 garlic cloves, minced

¼ pound lean ground beef

Salt and ground black pepper

¼ cup marinara sauce

Bring a large pot of water to a boil with a steamer insert. Halve the squash lengthwise and place in the steamer, cut side down. Cover and steam just until the squash is tender, 12 to 15 minutes. Remove from the steamer and set aside to cool slightly.

In a large nonstick skillet, heat the oil over medium-high heat. Add the onion and garlic and cook until the onion is translucent, about 3 minutes.

Add the beef, season with salt and pepper to taste, and cook, breaking up the meat with a spoon, until cooked through, about 10 minutes. Drain off any fat. Add the marinara and heat until warm.

With a fork, scrape the spaghetti squash flesh into long strands and place on a plate or in a pasta bowl. Top with the meat sauce.

Makes 1 serving

SALISBURY TURKEY

Nutrition per serving: Calories: 281 • Protein: 35 g • Carbs: 7 g • Fat: 13 g

This dish will make you forget bad cafeteria Salisbury steaks forever because this version is full of peppers and onions, which makes it sweet and juicy. Serve with vegetables and/or a mixed green salad.

¼ pound lean ground turkey

¼ red bell pepper, diced

¼ onion, diced

1 garlic clove, chopped

1 tablespoon balsamic vinegar

Salt and ground black pepper

Preheat the broiler. Line a broiler pan with foil.

In a large bowl, combine the turkey, bell pepper, onion, garlic, vinegar, and salt and black pepper to taste. Mix thoroughly and form into an oval patty about 2" thick.

Broil for 5 to 7 minutes per side, or until cooked through.

Makes 1 serving

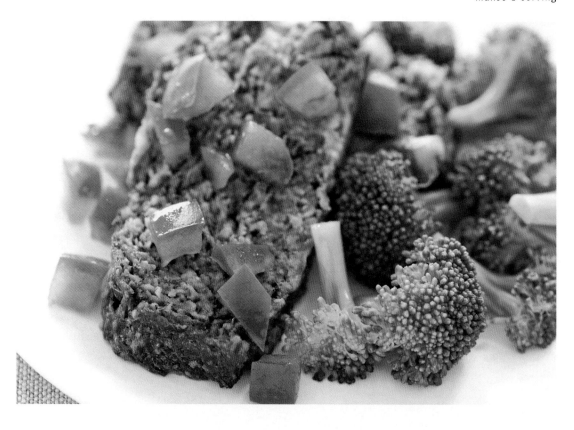

STUFFED PEPPERS

Nutrition per serving: Calories: 351 • Protein: 31 g • Carbs*: 18 g • Fat: 20 g

Using a pepper as the vehicle for a meat sauce instead of spaghetti not only cuts carbs, it also adds a great flavor dimension and looks cool on the plate.

  1 green bell pepper
  1 teaspoon olive oil
  ¼ onion, diced
  2 garlic cloves, minced
  ¼ pound lean ground beef
  ½ cup canned diced tomatoes
  Pinch of red-pepper flakes
  2 tablespoons shredded reduced-fat mozzarella cheese

Preheat the oven to 350°F.

Bring a medium saucepan of water to a boil. Cut off the stem and the top ¼" of the bell pepper and remove the ribs and seeds. Immerse the pepper in the boiling water and cook until it softens slightly. Remove the pepper from the water and set cut side down to drain.

In a large nonstick skillet, heat the oil over medium-high heat. Add the onion and garlic and cook until softened, about 3 minutes. Add the beef and cook, breaking up the meat with a spoon, until browned, 3 to 5 minutes. Drain off any fat. Stir in the tomatoes and pepper flakes and simmer for 3 to 5 minutes to thicken the sauce.

Cut a thin sliver off the bottom of the pepper to help it stand upright and place in a small baking dish. Fill it with the beef mixture, top with the cheese, and bake for 20 to 30 minutes, or until the pepper is tender and the cheese is melted.

Makes 1 serving

*Although this meal provides 18 grams of total carbs, 6 of those grams come from fiber, which means that you are really consuming only 12 grams of net carbs.

MINCED CHICKEN IN LETTUCE CUPS

Nutrition per serving: Calories: 235 • Protein: 28 g • Carbs: 14 g • Fat: 6g

Many restaurant chicken salads are actually full of carbs, with sugary dressings, croutons, and other no-nos. This one is pure protein and good veggies, with none of the carbs.

> 1 teaspoon olive oil
> 1 carrot, diced
> 2 tablespoons reduced-sodium soy sauce
> 4 ounces cooked chicken breast, finely chopped
> 1 scallion, sliced
> 3 Boston lettuce leaves

In a large nonstick skillet, heat the oil over medium-high heat. Add the carrot and cook for 1 minute. Add the soy sauce and cook, stirring occasionally, until the carrot is softened, about 3 minutes. Add the chicken and cook just to heat through. Stir in the scallion and remove from the heat. Spoon onto the lettuce leaves.

Makes 1 serving

SPICY BROILED SALMON

Nutrition per serving: Calories: 332 • Protein: 35 g • Carbs: 6 g • Fat: 18 g

Don't you just love a good piece of fish? This spicy salmon is rich in the essential fats you need for a lean and healthy body.

> ¼ cup fresh lime juice
> 2 garlic cloves, minced
> ¼ teaspoon cayenne pepper
> 6 ounces salmon fillet, skin removed

Preheat the broiler. Line a broiler pan with foil.

In a small bowl, whisk together the lime juice, garlic, and cayenne. Place the salmon on the broiler pan and top with the lime mixture. Broil for 5 to 6 minutes, or until the fish just flakes with a fork but is still moist.

Makes 1 serving

TURKEY CHILI

Nutrition per serving: Calories: 321• Protein: 38 g• Carbs: 37 g• Fat: 2.5 g

This turkey chili may be lean, but it has plenty of heart. If only your favorite football team could say the same. Ah, Sundays.

  1 teaspoon olive oil

  1 onion, diced

  2 garlic cloves, minced

  1 pound extra-lean ground turkey breast

  Salt and ground black pepper

  2 cans (14.5 ounces each) diced tomatoes

  1 can (15.25 ounces) kidney beans, rinsed and drained

  1 can (6 ounces) tomato paste

  1 tablespoon chili powder

  Hot sauce (optional)

In a large nonstick skillet, heat the oil over medium-high heat. Add the onion, garlic, turkey, and salt and pepper to taste. Cook, breaking up the turkey with a spoon, until browned, 3 to 5 minutes.

Add the tomatoes, beans, tomato paste, and chili powder and mix well. Bring to a simmer and cook over low heat until thickened, about 30 minutes. Serve with hot sauce, if desired.

Makes 4 servings

CHICKEN WITH EGG NOODLES

Nutrition per serving: Calories: 448 • Protein: 51 g • Carbs: 44 g • Fat: 6 g

Is there any food more versatile than chicken? Here we get it acquainted with whole wheat egg noodles, which introduces you to a whole new kind of taste. Oh, by the way, it's high in carbs and low in fat.

1¼ cups cooked whole wheat egg noodles

½ cup zucchini, steamed

¼ cup fat-free ricotta cheese

½ teaspoon dried oregano

Salt and ground black pepper

4 ounces cooked chicken breast, shredded

In a medium bowl, combine the egg noodles, zucchini, ricotta, and oregano. Season with salt and pepper to taste, and toss to combine. Serve topped with the chicken.

Makes 1 serving

LEMON-CHICKEN RISOTTO

Nutrition per serving: Calories: 342 • Protein: 33 g • Carbs: 42 g • Fat: 4 g

Add a little of that Old World Italian flavor to kick-start a lazy Sunday afternoon. This serves 4, so invite some buddies over. Still a whole lot of football left to watch.

1 teaspoon olive oil

1 pound boneless, skinless chicken breast, cubed

1 onion, diced

Pinch of red-pepper flakes

1 cup Arborio rice

½ cup fresh lemon juice

2 cups low-sodium chicken broth

¼ cup chopped fresh basil

¼ cup grated Parmesan cheese

In a large nonstick skillet, heat the oil over medium-high heat. Add the chicken and cook, stirring occasionally, until browned and cooked through, about 8 minutes. Transfer the chicken to a plate.

Add the onion, pepper flakes, and rice to the skillet. Stir to coat the rice with the pan drippings. Add the lemon juice and simmer until absorbed. Add the broth ½ cup at a time, stirring frequently after each addition until the liquid is absorbed. Cook until the rice is tender, about 30 minutes. Mix in the basil and cheese. Serve the risotto topped with the chicken.

Makes 4 servings

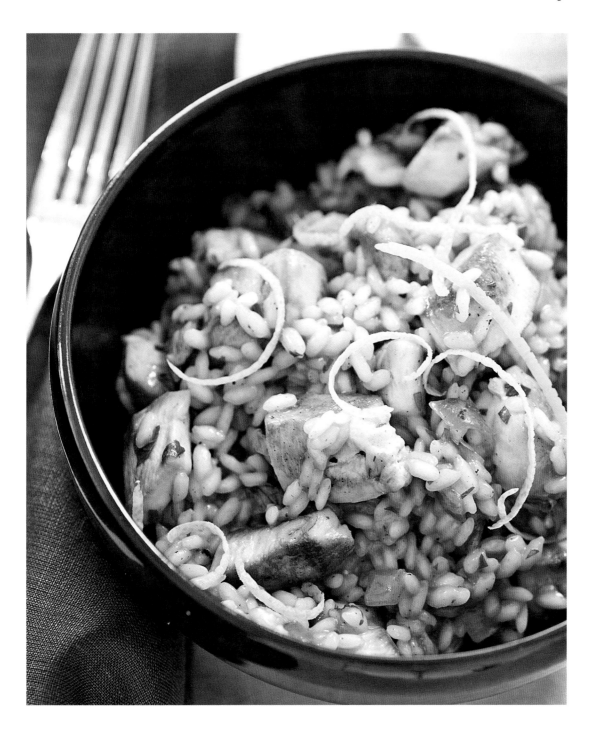

SNACKS

PEANUT BUTTER PUDDING

Nutrition per serving: Calories: 265 • Protein: 28 g • Carbs: 12 g • Fat: 13 g

Just like Grandma used to make, except it will give you the protein and healthy fats you need to keep your metabolic rate up and your hunger in check. Take that, cravings.

1 tablespoon peanut butter
1 teaspoon honey
1 cup 2% plain Greek yogurt

Stir the peanut butter and honey into the yogurt.

Makes 1 serving

CRUNCHY COTTAGE CHEESE

Nutrition per serving: Calories: 141 • Protein: 16 g • Carbs: 10 g • Fat: 4 g

This protein powerhouse not only delivers slow-digesting protein to help your muscles recover from workouts, it also provides essential fats to enhance fat loss and speed up recovery.

½ cup 2% cottage cheese
¼ cup blueberries or strawberries
1 teaspoon flaxseed, toasted

In a small bowl, combine the cottage cheese, berries, and flaxseed.

Makes 1 serving

CRABBY DEVILED EGGS

Nutrition per serving: Calories: 255 • Protein: 26 g • Carbs: 1 g • Fat: 15 g

Having a devil of a time coming up with new ways to turn hard-boiled eggs into treats that deliver big-time protein? Not anymore you aren't.

3 large eggs, hard-boiled

3 ounces canned lump crabmeat, drained

½ celery rib, finely minced

1 tablespoon light mayonnaise

1 teaspoon Dijon mustard

Salt and ground black pepper

Hot sauce (optional)

Halve the eggs lengthwise. Discard 1 yolk and place the remaining 2 yolks in a bowl. Add the crab, celery, mayonnaise, and mustard and mix thoroughly. Fill the egg-white halves with the crab mixture. Season with salt and pepper to taste and hot sauce (if desired).

Makes 1 serving

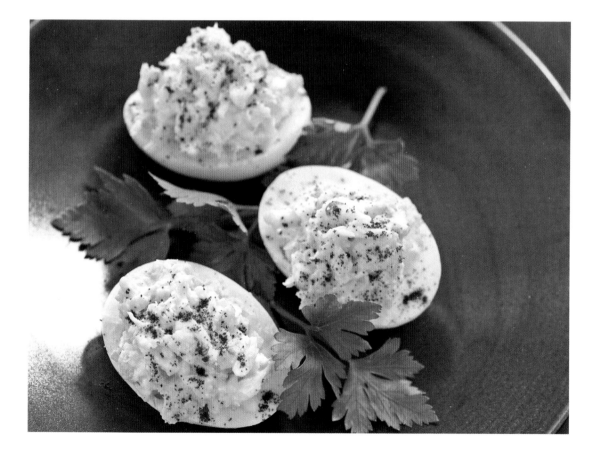

ONION DIP

Nutrition per serving: Calories: 150 • Protein: 20 g • Carbs: 9 g • Fat: 5 g

This may seem like you are dipping into decadence, but it's really a high-protein snack.

- 1 cup 2% plain Greek yogurt
- 1 teaspoon garlic salt
- 1 teaspoon onion powder
- 1 tablespoon chopped fresh chives
- 1 cup mixed raw vegetables (carrots, celery, broccoli, sliced bell peppers)

In a medium bowl, combine the yogurt, garlic salt, onion powder, and chives and mix well. Serve the dip with the veggies for dunking.

Makes 1 serving

WHOLE WHEAT TORTILLA CHIPS AND CREAM CHEESE DIP

Nutrition per serving: Calories: 117 • Protein: 14 g • Carbs: 15 g • Fat: 2 g

You want amazing? This low-calorie snack still contains 14 grams of protein. It'll have your taste buds jumping.

- 1 low-carb whole wheat tortilla (8")
- 2 ounces (4 tablespoons) fat-free cream cheese
- 1 tablespoon 1% milk
- 1 teaspoon garlic salt
- 2 tablespoons chopped fresh chives

Preheat the oven to 350°F. Slice the tortilla into eighths and place on a baking sheet. Bake until slightly browned and crunchy.

Meanwhile, in a small bowl, stir the cream cheese and milk together until smooth. Stir in the garlic salt and chives. Serve the chips with the dip.

Makes 1 serving

WORKOUT LOG: PHASE 1/Week 1

Exercise	Sets	Reps	Day 1	Day 2	Day 3	Day 4	Day 5	Day 6
Leg Press	2	12–15		C		C		C
Leg Extension	2	12–15		A		A		A
Lying Leg Curl	2	12–15		R		R		R
Lat Pulldown	2	12–15		D		D		D
Machine Chest Press	2	12–15		I		I		I
Machine Row	2	12–15		O		O		O
Overhead Machine Press	2	12–15						
Machine Preacher Curl	2	12–15						
Cable Pressdown	2	12–15						
Standing Calf Raise	2	12–15						
Crunch	2	12–15						

20-minute steady-state cardio workout (slow and easy)

WORKOUT LOG: PHASE 1/Week 2

Exercise	Sets	Reps	Day 1	Day 2	Day 3	Day 4	Day 5	Day 6
Leg Press	2	12–15		C		C		C
Leg Extension	2	12–15		A		A		A
Lying Leg Curl	2	12–15		R		R		R
Lat Pulldown	2	12–15		D		D		D
Machine Chest Press	2	12–15		I		I		I
Machine Row	2	12–15		O		O		O
Overhead Machine Press	2	12–15						
Machine Preacher Curl	2	12–15						
Cable Pressdown	2	12–15						
Standing Calf Raise	2	12–15						
Crunch	2	12–15						

20-minute steady-state cardio workout (slow and easy)
Rest 1 minute between sets; does not include warmup sets.

WORKOUT LOG: PHASE 2/Weeks 3 and 4

DAY 1: Upper Body Exercises	Sets	Reps	Weight Week 3	Weight Week 4
Smith Bench Press	3	8–12		
Seated Cable Row	3	8–12		
Standing Overhead Press	2	8–12		
Barbell Curl	3	8–12		
Cable Pressdown	3	8–12		
Cable Crunch	3	8–12		
30-minute steady-state workout (slow and easy)				

DAY 2: Lower Body Exercises	Sets	Reps	Weight Week 3	Weight Week 4
Smith Squat	3	8–12		
Leg Press	3	8–12		
Dumbbell Stepup	2	8–12		
Leg Extension	3	8–12		
Barbell Lunge	3	8–12		
Lying Leg Curl	3	8–12		
Seated Calf Raise	2	8–12		
20-minute interval cardio workout				

DAY 3: REST

DAY 4: Upper Body Exercises	Sets	Reps	Weight Week 3	Weight Week 4
Smith Bench Press	3	8–12		
Seated Cable Row	3	8–12		
Standing Overhead Press	2	8–12		
Barbell Curl	3	8–12		
Cable Pressdown	3	8–12		
Cable Crunch	3	8–12		
30-minute steady-state workout (slow and easy)				

DAY 5: Lower Exercises	Sets	Reps	Weight Week 3	Weight Week 4
Smith Squat	3	8–12		
Leg Press	3	8–12		
Dumbbell Stepup	2	8–12		
Leg Extension	3	8–12		
Barbell Lunge	3	8–12		
Lying Leg Curl	3	8–12		
Seated Calf Raise	2	8–12		
20-minute interval cardio workout				
In all workouts, rest 1 minute between sets; does not include warmup sets.				

DAYS 6 and 7: REST

WORKOUT LOG: PHASE 3/Weeks 5 and 6

DAY 1: Chest, Shoulders, Triceps Exercises	Sets	Reps	Weight Week 5	Weight Week 6
Dumbbell Bench Press	3	8–12		
Incline Cable Fly	3	8–12		
Weighted Dip	2	8–12		
Upright Row	3	8–12		
Seated Overhead Dumbbell Press	3	8–12		
Cable Lateral Raise	2	8–12		
Cable Kickback	3	8–12		
Reverse-Grip Pressdown	3	8–12		
Bench Dip	2	8–12		
Overhead Cable Extension	2	8–12		
35-minute interval cardio workout				

DAY 2: Legs Exercises	Sets	Reps	Weight Week 5	Weight Week 6
Barbell Squat	3	8–12		
Leg Press	3	8–12		
Hack Squat	2	8–12		
Leg Extension	3	8–12		
Barbell Lunge	3	8–12		
Lying Leg Curl	3	8–12		
Standing Calf Raise	2	8–12		
Seated Calf Raise	2	8–12		
25-minute steady-state cardio workout				

DAY 3: Back, Biceps, Abs, Calves Exercises	Sets	Reps	Weight Week 5	Weight Week 6
Straight-Arm Pulldown	3	8–12		
Dumbbell Pullover	3	8–12		
Seated Cable Row	3	8–12		
Dumbbell Curl	3	8–12		
Incline Dumbbell Curl	2	8–12		
Dumbbell Preacher Curl	2	8–12		
Hanging Leg Raise	3	to failure		
Weighted Crunch	3	8–12		
Standing Calf Raise	3	8–12		

DAY 4: REST

WORKOUT LOG: PHASE 3–cont.

DAY 5: Chest, Shoulders, Triceps Exercises	Sets	Reps	Weight Week 5	Weight Week 6
Dumbbell Bench Press	3	8–12		
Incline Cable Fly	3	8–12		
Weighted Dip	2	8–12		
Upright Row	3	8–12		
Seated Overhead Dumbbell Press	3	8–12		
Cable Lateral Raise	2	8–12		
Cable Kickback	3	8–12		
Reverse-Grip Pressdown	3	8–12		
Bench Dip	2	8–12		
Overhead Cable Extension	2	8–12		
35-minute interval cardio workout				

DAY 6: Legs Exercises	Sets	Reps	Weight Week 5	Weight Week 6
Barbell Squat	3	8–12		
Leg Press	3	8–12		
Hack Squat	2	8–12		
Leg Extension	3	8–12		
Barbell Lunge	3	8–12		
Lying Leg Curl	3	8–12		
Standing Calf Raise	2	8–12		
Seated Calf Raise	2	8–12		
25-minute steady-state cardio workout				

Rest 1½ minutes between all sets in all workouts; does not include warmup sets.

DAY 7: Back, Biceps, Abs, Calves Exercises	Sets	Reps	Weight Week 5	Weight Week 6
Straight-Arm Pulldown	3	8–12		
Dumbbell Pullover	3	8–12		
Seated Cable Row	3	8–12		
Dumbbell Curl	3	8–12		
Incline Dumbbell Curl	2	8–12		
Dumbbell Preacher Curl	2	8–12		
Hanging Leg Raise	3	to failure		
Weighted Crunch	3	8–12		
Standing Calf Raise	3	8–12		

WORKOUT LOG: PHASE 4/Weeks 7 and 8

DAY 1: Chest, Shoulders, Triceps, Abs Exercises	Sets	Reps	Weight Week 7	Weight Week 8
Incline Bench Press*	4	12, 12, 8, 8		
Flat-Bench Dumbbell Fly	3	12, 10, 8		
Bench Dip	3	12, 10, 8		
Overhead Dumbbell Press*	4	12, 12, 6, 6		
Upright Row	3	8, 6, 6		
Cable Lateral Raise	3	12, 12, 12		
Close-Grip Bench Press	3	12, 12, 12		
Rope Pressdown*	3	15, 10, 8		
Cable Crunch	3	To failure		
superset with				
Hanging Leg Raise	3	To failure		
35-minute interval cardio workout				

DAY 2: Legs, Calves, Back, Biceps, Forearms, Abs Exercises	Sets	Reps	Weight Week 7	Weight Week 8
Leg Press*	4	12, 12, 8, 6		
Leg Extension	3	10, 10, 8		
Lying Leg Curl	3	10, 10, 8		
Romanian Deadlift	3	10, 10, 8		
Seated Calf Raise	4	25, 25, 12, 12		
Lat Pulldown*	3	12, 8, 8		
Seated Cable Row (wide grip)	3	12, 12, 12		
Dumbbell Row	3	12, 12, 12		
Barbell Curl*	4	12, 10, 8, 6		
Incline Dumbbell Curl	3	10, 10, 8		
One-Arm Cable Curl	3	10, 10, 8		
Dumbbell Wrist Curl*	3	12, 10, 10		
Hanging Knee Raise	3	To failure		
Crunch (page 43)	2	15, 15		
25-minute steady-state cardio workout				

DAY 3: REST

WORKOUT LOG: PHASE 4—cont.

DAY 4: Chest, Shoulders, Traps, Triceps, Abs Exercises	Sets	Reps	Weight Week 7	Weight Week 8
Decline Bench Press*	3	12, 10, 8		
Dumbbell Bench Press	3	10, 8, 6		
Pec-Deck Fly	3	10, 8, 6		
Overhead Machine Press*	4	12, 10, 8, 6		
Dumbbell Lateral Raise	3	10, 8, 6		
Dumbbell Front Raise	3	10, 10, 10		
Barbell Shrug	3	6, 6, 6		
Straight-Bar Cable Pressdown*	3	10, 10, 8		
Overhead Cable Extension	3	10, 8, 6		
Weighted Dip (page 59)	3	10, 8, 6		
Hanging Knee Raise	3	To failure		
Weighted Crunch	2	To failure		
35-minute interval cardio workout				

DAY 5: REST

DAY 6: Legs, Back, Biceps, Abs Exercises	Sets	Reps	Weight Week 7	Weight Week 8
Smith Squat	4	10, 10, 6, 6		
Walking Lunge	3	10, 10, 8		
Lying Leg Curl	3	10, 10, 8		
Romanian Deadlift	3	10, 10, 8		
Standing Calf Raise*	3	10, 12, 15		
Bent-Over Barbell Row	3	10, 8, 6		
Seated Cable Row	3	10, 8, 6		
Lat Pulldown (underhand grip)	3	12, 12, 12		
Dumbbell Curl*	4	10, 8, 6, 6		
Dumbbell Preacher Curl	3	10, 8, 6		
Crunch	3	To failure		
Hanging Leg Raise	3	To failure		
25-minute steady-state cardio workout				

*Perform as a drop set; the reps listed are the number you do on that first set before you lighten the weight. On that first drop, continue until muscle failure. Rest 2 minutes between drop sets and 1 minute between all other sets.

DAY 7: REST

WORKOUT LOG: PHASE 5/Platinum Advanced

DAY 1: Arms Exercises	Sets	Reps	Time	Weight
Barbell Curl	3	6, 8, 25		
Jump Rope			1 minute	
Preacher Curl	3	6, 8, 25		
Jump Squat			1 minute	
Incline Cable Curl	3	6, 8, 25		
Jump Rope			1 minute	
Lying Triceps Extension	3	6, 8, 25		
Jump Squat			1 minute	
Rope Pressdown	3	6, 8, 25		
Jump Rope			1 minute	
Overhead Dumbbell Extension	3	6, 8, 25		
Jump Squat			1 minute	

DAY 2: Legs Exercises	Sets	Reps	Time	Weight
Barbell Squat	3	6, 8, 25		
Lateral Box Hops			1 minute	
Hack Squat	3	6, 8, 25		
Split-Jump Squat			1 minute	
Leg Extension	3	6, 8, 25		
Lateral Box Hops			1 minute	
Romanian Deadlift	3	6, 8, 25		
Split-Jump Squat			1 minute	
Seated Leg Curl	3	6, 8, 25		
Lateral Box Hops			1 minute	
Standing Calf Raise	3	6, 8, 25		
Split-Jump Squat			1 minute	
Seated Calf Raise	3	6, 8, 25		
Lateral Box Hops			1 minute	

*Rest 1 minute between sets. Once you've completed all 3 sets of an exercise, perform 1 minute of activity, as indicated.

DAY 3: Cardio and Abs Exercises	Sets	Reps	Time	Weight
Hanging Knee Raise	3	To failure		
Crunch	3	To failure		
Knee-Ins	3	To failure		
Standing Calf Raise (page 42)	3	To failure		
Seated Calf Raise (page 54)	3	To failure		

Cardio: Start workout with a bout on the treadmill, stairclimber, or step mill for 1 full hour.

WORKOUT LOG: PHASE 5—cont.

DAY 4: Chest, Shoulders Exercises	Sets	Reps	Time	Weight
Incline Bench Press	3	6, 8, 25		
Jump Rope			1 minute	
Incline Cable Fly	3	6, 8, 25		
Jump Squat			1 minute	
Smith Bench Press	3	6, 8, 25		
Jump Rope			1 minute	
Incline-Bench Cable Fly	3	6, 8, 25		
Jump Squat			1 minute	
Decline Press	3	6, 8, 25		
Jump Rope			1 minute	
Standing Overhead Press	3	6, 8, 25		
Jump Squat			1 minute	
Cable Lateral Raise	3	6, 8, 25		
Jump Rope			1 minute	
Bent-Over Cable Lateral Raise	3	6, 8, 25		
Jump Squat			1 minute	

DAY 5: Back, Traps Exercises	Sets	Reps	Time	Weight
Deadlift	3	6, 8, 25		
Lateral Box Hops			1 minute	
Dumbbell Row	3	6, 8, 25		
Split-Jump Squat			1 minute	
Reverse-Grip Lat Pulldown	3	6, 8, 25		
Lateral Box Hops			1 minute	
Seated Cable Row (wide grip)	3	6, 8, 25		
Split-Jump Squat			1 minute	
Barbell Shrug	3	6, 8, 25		
Lateral Box Hops			1 minute	
Dumbbell Shrug	3	6, 8, 25		
Split-Jump Squat			1 minute	
Pullup	3	To failure		

Rest 1 minute between sets. Once you've completed all 3 sets of an exercise, perform 1 minute of activity, as indicated.

DAY 6: Cardio, Abs, Calves Exercise	Sets	Reps	Time	Weight
Hanging Knee Raise	3	To failure		
Machine Crunch	3	10–12		
Standing Calf Raise	3	20		
Seated Calf Raise	3	20		

Cardio: Precede abs and calves with a 1-hour session on the treadmill or stairclimber at a steady pace.
Rest 1 minute between sets in all workouts.

ACKNOWLEDGMENTS

First and foremost, I would like to thank GOD for all he's done and continues to do in my life. I would like to thank my wife, Simone, and my kids, Najee, Italia, Samaria, and Nina, for all their love and support; my mom, Ondrea; Aunt Cammy; DJ Cut Creator, my man from day 1; Claudine 24/7 Joseph, for always getting it done; Chris Lighty; David "Scooter" Honig; Jason "The Alchemist" Barrett; Jason Sloane; A. J. Brandenstein; Michael Hertz; David Garelik; Leslie Moonves; Nina Tassler; Nancy Tellem; Jack Sussman; David Brownfield; George Schweitzer; Katie Barker; Kristen Hall; David Stapf; Shane Brennan; R. Scott Gemmill; John P. Kousakis; Chris O'Donnell; Linda Hunt; Daniela Ruah; Peter Cambor; Barrett Foa; Adam Jamal Craig; Jonathan Tisch; Matt Blank; Stewart Rahr; Monica Morrow; Leisa Balfour; Richard "Rich4Life" Weitz, for believing; Cara Lewis; my mentor the Honorable Reverend Floyd H. Flake, D. Min. Pastor; the Reverend M. Elaine Flake, D. Min. Co-Pastor; my friend Bishop Kenneth C. and Togetta Ulmer; Ken Erhlich; Ron Gabrisko; Chris Burgoyne; Kevin Smith; Aaron Speiser; Chanda Counts; Marc Gerald; Haim Dabah; Keesha Johnson; Rhett Usry; Chris Palmer; Jim Stoppani; Boomdizzle.com; Simone I. Smith Jewelry; designer Chris Rhoads and the team at Rodale; CBS; CBS Television Studios; Paramount.

—LL COOL J

I would like to dedicate my portion of the book to my mom, Frances Honig. My love and thanks to my second mom, Arlyne Smith, a warrior who made it better for all she came in contact with. To LL Cool J, who has allowed me to be part of his team for the past 9 years, I thank you. My team, Jim Stoppani, Chris Palmer, Claudine Joseph, and Heather Downey, our female model. Pam Krauss and the team from Rodale, especially Chris Rhoads for all his time and patience, thank you for your commitment.

To Debbie Smith for just being honest and loyal; my family, Vic and Leslie Honig, and their children Marissa, Michael, Megan, and Maddy; my friend Eddie O'Boyle, who always had faith in me; Brian Daughtry; Jeff Frankel; Paul Holtzman; Eddie Guyton; Peter G; Bobby Podolsky; Chris Aceto; Dr. Laurence Spier; Chris O'Boyle; Rich McCarthy; Brian Killingsworth; Dr. Brownstein; James Forgione; Scott Campbell; Menorah Manor; and David Buer, my partner in SXFitness, for all his inspiration and ideas. Jimmy Pena for his sincerity and professionalism; Barry Schneider for all his support and friendship. I thank you all.

—David "Scooter" Honig

INDEX

Boldface page references indicate photographs. <u>Underscored</u> references indicate boxed text.